Staying Motivated
Daily Rituals to Stay Motivated!
By Kevin James Joseph McNamara

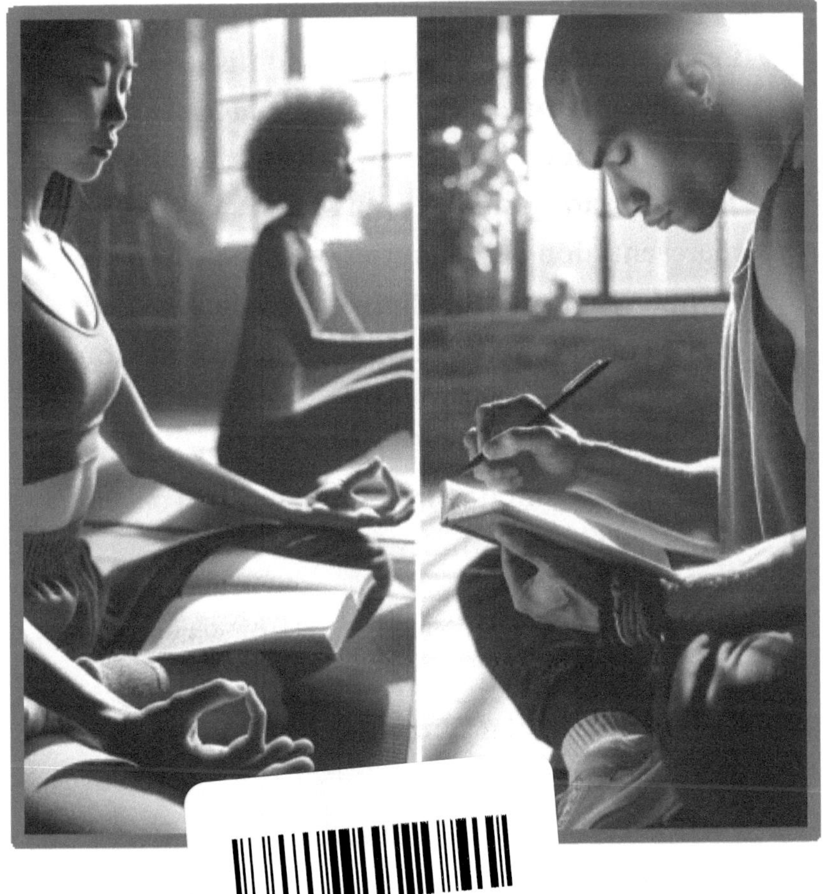

Published By Kevin James Joseph McNamara

~ ~ ~

this material, which is provided "as is," and without warranties.

As always, the advice of a competent professional should be sought. The author and publisher do not warrant the performance, effectiveness or applicability of any sites listed or linked to in this eBook. All links are for information purposes only and are not warranted for content, accuracy or any other implied or explicit purpose.

Table of Contents

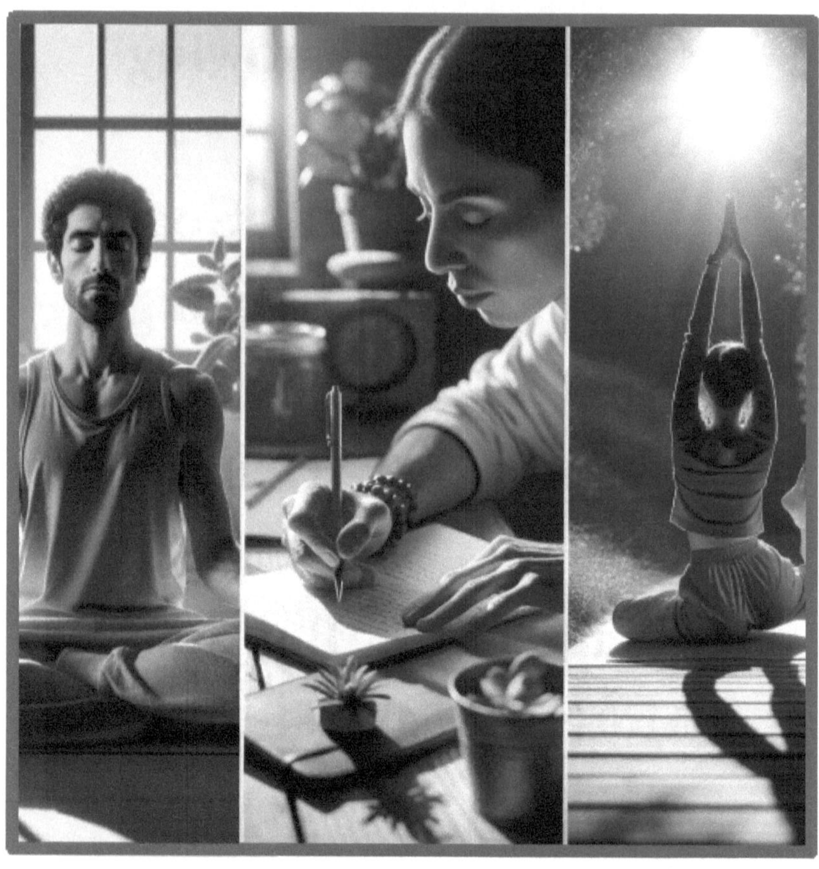

Chapter 1 – Introduction

Motivation is what keeps us going. It is the reason people succeed and the reason people fail. Motivation is the drive someone has to complete a task. The ingredients of motivation are combined with many factors which include simplicity, attitude, the people you hang around, the way you think, knowing yourself, helping other people and so much more.

The purpose of this e-book is to take you through methods you can practice on a daily basis to remain motivated. These techniques can help you feel better about yourself in everything you do. You can take these methods with you when you go to work and when you are at home.

Motivation is the spark everyone needs to make it throughout the day, to set and meet goals, and more. Without motivation, you will fail. When you have apathy toward something, you are not motivated because you could not care either way. This is the worst attitude you can have because it is not negative either. Someone who feels this way is not capable of achieving anything because they do not care if they do or not. If you are feeling this way, this e-book is exactly what you need to help you overcome your attitude and begin feeling motivated again.

When you know how to remain motivated with yourself, you can also help others because your attitude will be contagious. When you practice daily motivational techniques, eventually, they will come to you naturally. At first, some of these methods may be difficult for you to do or to remember. It will take time for you to begin to naturally practice and follow these techniques.

The key to staying motivated is understanding what drives you. Once you discover what fuels your passion, it becomes easier to maintain your focus and achieve your goals. This e-book will guide you through various strategies to find your motivation and keep it alive.

One crucial aspect of motivation is setting clear and achievable goals. When you have a specific target in mind, it gives you a sense of direction and purpose. This e-book will provide you with tips on how to set effective goals and how to break them down into manageable steps.

Another important factor in staying motivated is maintaining a positive mindset. Your thoughts have a significant impact on your feelings and actions. This e-book will offer techniques to cultivate a positive attitude and to overcome negative thinking patterns that may hinder your progress.

Surrounding yourself with supportive people is also vital for maintaining motivation. The right environment can inspire and encourage you to keep moving forward. This e-book will discuss the importance of building a positive support system and how to deal with negativity from others.

In addition to these strategies, this e-book will cover various topics such as time management, stress management, and the power of visualization. By implementing these techniques, you can enhance your motivation and increase your chances of success in all areas of your life.

Finally, this e-book will emphasize the importance of self-care and balance. Taking care of your physical and mental well-being is essential for sustaining motivation over the long term. You will learn how to incorporate healthy habits into your daily routine and how to find a balance between work and relaxation.

By the end of this e-book, you will have a comprehensive understanding of motivation and the tools needed to stay motivated. Whether you are looking to achieve personal or professional goals, the insights and techniques provided in this e-book will empower you to take control of your life and reach your full potential.

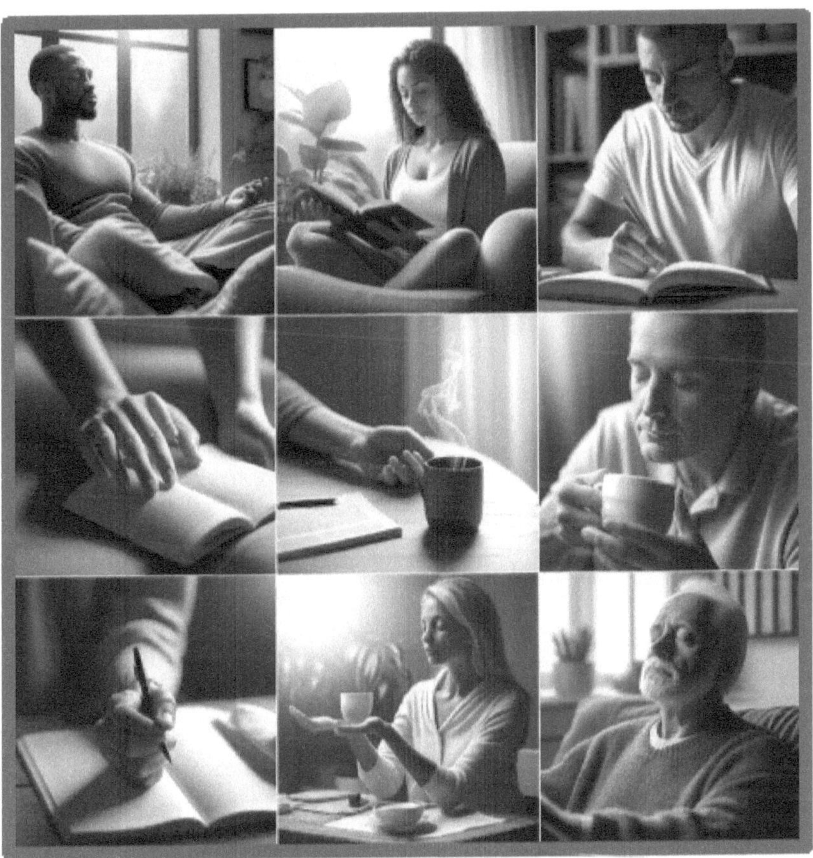

Chapter 2 – Keeping It Simple

When thinking about motivation, the first thing you need to do is create your space around you at work and at home. This space needs to remain simple and positive. The things around you have a lot to do with the way you feel and if you are motivated or stuck in a funk.

Your office space should contain and display items that make you feel positive about life and about reaching goals. If you have goals and things you would like to do, it might be a good idea to post these things on the wall of your office or your cubicle. This way, you have a constant reminder of the things you would eventually like to do.

Only you know where you would like to be in the future. You should create your space as a constant and positive reminder that you are working to get there. Create a positive atmosphere around you no matter where you are. This also includes the car you drive. If you spend many hours in the car commuting every day, make it a positive space. This means clean it up. Do not drive around a depressing vehicle that is full of trash and paperwork. Get your car detailed and begin to take care of it. You would be surprised how good you will feel when you clean up your car.

A clean home and clean office space make a really big deal when you need motivation. If you find yourself sitting in mounds of paperwork, you might have the attitude you are never going to complete the things you need done. A messy workspace can be frustrating and depressing. It may cause you to procrastinate and even be disorganized with your thoughts as well as your work.

A messy and dirty home can be depressing and disabling. Many people will sit around procrastinating for hours in a messy home. It is amazing how good a clean home can make you feel. The best thing you can do is clean up your home. You will feel great and ready to take on anything. Get rid of those clothes which have been sitting in the closet for years that you have not worn once. Clean out the mess in the shed and the garage. Do not just wipe down the counters and do the dishes. A clean house means creating a new space that is positive and ready for the new to come into your home. Get rid of all of the old.

The space you spend your time in includes your car, home, and the office space you work in. It has a lot to do with the way you feel and the attitude you have when you wake up in the morning. Clean up the spaces you live in and make a positive atmosphere for you to enjoy and have a good day. You will finally see the goals as achievable rather than sit around thinking about them.

Creating a simple and organized environment is crucial for maintaining motivation. Clutter and chaos can be overwhelming and distracting, making it difficult to focus on your goals. By simplifying your surroundings, you can reduce stress and increase your productivity.

One way to simplify your life is to adopt a minimalist approach. This does not mean you have to get rid of everything you own, but rather focus on keeping only what is necessary and meaningful. By decluttering your space, you can create a more peaceful and efficient environment.

In addition to physical clutter, it is important to address mental clutter as well. This includes negative thoughts, unnecessary worries, and unproductive habits. By practicing mindfulness and positive thinking, you can clear your mind and stay focused on your goals.

Another aspect of keeping it simple is to establish routines and systems that work for you. Whether it is a morning routine that sets the tone for your day or a system for organizing your tasks, having a consistent approach can help you stay on track and reduce decision fatigue.

Finally, remember that simplicity is not about perfection. It is about making your life easier and more enjoyable. Do not be afraid to make changes and adjustments as needed. The goal is to find a balance that allows you to be productive and motivated without feeling overwhelmed.

By embracing simplicity in your life, you can create a positive and supportive environment that encourages motivation and success. Whether you are working towards personal or professional goals, a simple and organized approach can help you stay focused and achieve your aspirations.

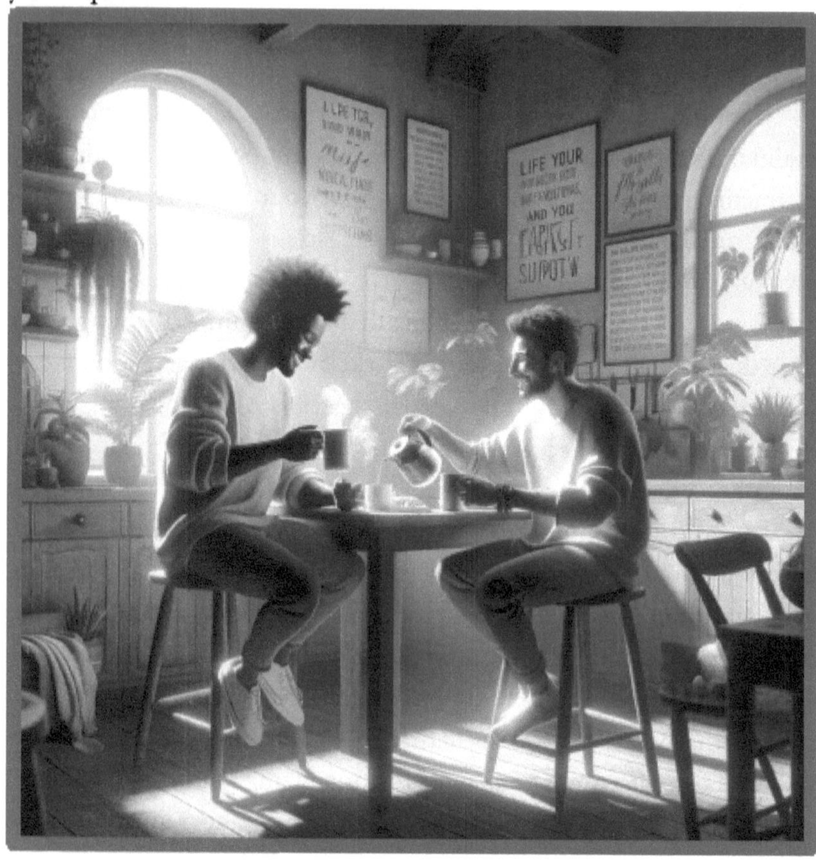

Chapter 3 – Keeping Good Company

Hanging out with positive people is one of the best ways to be motivated. You should talk to someone positive at least once a day. Many of the ways you can have a positive encounter with people include in person, over the phone, and over the computer. Try to make this a habit on a daily basis.

Some people are not very social. They might go days without talking to others. This is very unhealthy. If you are one of these people who is not a very social person and find that you do not have many encounters with others, you probably also are not too motivated to succeed also. This does not mean you have to be a social bug. What this means is that you need to feed your need for positive interaction. You do not have to see the other person either. There are techniques you can practice to encounter others positively without even seeing them in person. How you do these things is up to you, but this is especially important.

Keeping good company means hanging out with others who are supportive of you and your goals for life. You want people to support you and believe in you too. If you have goals to be successful with your own gardening company, you should spend time together with people who are supportive. If you are around people who are negative about your endeavors and unsupportive you will not feel good about it at all. Cut the negativity out. If these people are family members it could be the most difficult decision you ever made. However, it will be the best thing you can do for you. If people are not supportive or positive, then cut them out.

The most common way you can have an encounter with someone on a daily basis is to talk to people. You should have regular encounters with positive people. The best way to start your day is to have coffee every morning with a positive person. If you live near your best friend who is a coffee drinker, then you can plan to leave for work earlier every day and have coffee at their house or have them come over. This is an excellent way to start your day and put you in a great mood for work. You will already start the social side of you so when you get to work you will not feel like such a grouch.

If you do not have time in the mornings to meet with someone or any other time of day you should try to find the time to talk to someone on the phone. You might have a best friend you can call and talk to or a family member. Be sure the person is someone that makes you feel good about yourself and life.

If you do not like to talk on the phone and you do not have time to stop by and talk to someone every day, then you might consider the Internet your best option. Many people use this method as a way to keep good company. When you go online you can join a chat room for just about anything today. There are millions of chat rooms all over the web. Be sure to pick a chat room that is about something you feel good about. For instance, if you have a goal to do something you might join a group with others who are working toward the same goal. This is an exceptionally good way to boost your positive attitude and motivate you to work toward that goal.

Negativity can almost be infectious in some situations. You want to be sure the people you are talking to are positive. If the person you choose to hang out with is a negative person who is always complaining and who sees the negative side of everything, they might not be who you want to help you become motivated. Negativity will only bring you down and cause you to be negative too.

In addition to surrounding yourself with positive people, it is important to actively seek out inspiration. This can come in the form of books, podcasts, motivational speakers, or even uplifting music. By exposing yourself to inspiring content, you can fuel your motivation and maintain a positive mindset.

Another key aspect of keeping good company is to engage in activities that bring you joy and fulfillment. Whether it is pursuing a hobby, volunteering for a cause you care about, or simply spending time in nature, doing things that make you happy can boost your motivation and overall well-being.

It is also crucial to be mindful of the influence of social media on your motivation. While it can be a great tool for connecting with like-minded individuals and finding inspiration, it can also lead to comparison and negativity. Be selective about who you follow and make sure your social media feed is a source of positivity and encouragement.

Building a supportive network is another important aspect of keeping good company. This can include mentors, coaches, or accountability partners who can provide guidance, feedback, and encouragement as you work towards your goals. Having someone to share your successes and challenges with can be incredibly motivating.

Finally, remember that keeping good company is a two-way street. Be the positive influence and support for others that you seek for yourself. By being a source of encouragement and inspiration to those around you, you not only help others but also reinforce your own motivation and positivity.

By prioritizing positive interactions, seeking inspiration, engaging in fulfilling activities, being mindful of social media, building a supportive network, and being a positive influence, you can create an environment that fosters motivation and success. Surrounding yourself with good company is a powerful way to stay motivated and achieve your goals.

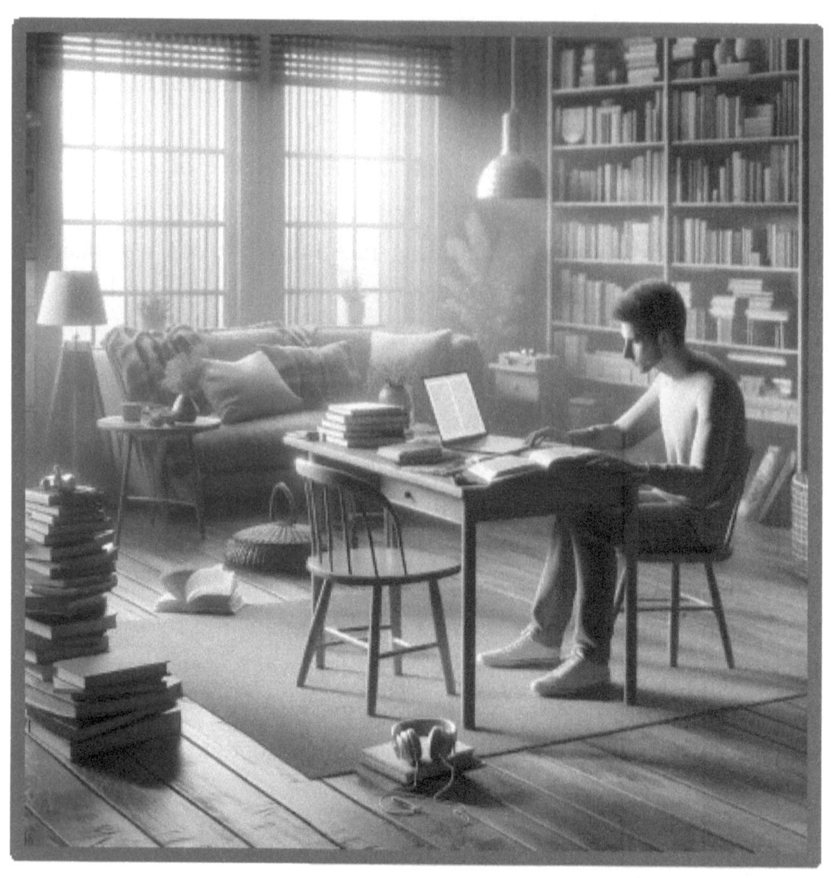

Chapter 4 – Continuous Learning

Learning promotes growth. It is healthy for the brain, and you are never too old to learn something new. Every day you should try to learn something new. The best ways to do this is through reading and listening.

If you are often not motivated to begin new projects or to take on new things you should increase your learning. You do not have to be an avid reader and take on novels, but you should read. Reading is good for the brain, and it is stimulating for the mind. Continuously learning new things will help you become open to take on things you did not think you could do before.

A morning newspaper is a common way some people like to stimulate their brain. They might like to cuddle up with the paper and their coffee before they begin their long day or even read the newspaper every night before you go to bed. This is an excellent habit to get into.

Reading the newspaper can be difficult for some people. You might not like the newspaper because of the ink, or you believe in recycling, and you are against the abundance of newspapers being printed. You do not have to read the newspaper. You can read the news online every day on your computer. You do not have to be on a news site, but you can read anything that interests you. Maybe you would like to learn a new skill. You can go to a site that focuses on this skill and read a little bit every day.

Reading is not the only thing you can do to continuously be learning. If you do not have time to read or if you do not like to read there are other ways you can learn. Many people who have long commutes often listen to audio CD's. Some people learn a different language or listen to a novel. There are many different things you can listen to any time of day.

Listening can also extend to your television while you are getting ready for work. You might choose to turn on the news and listen to the news every morning. You can listen to a cooking channel or public radio. You do not have to read if you are not a big reader.

Listening to your friends, family, and other people is another important aspect you need to focus on to remain motivated. When you listen to others, they will want to be around you because they will know what they say means something to you and you will learn. You will feel good about yourself as you respect others, which will build motivation.

Continuous learning is extremely important to motivation. Every day you should maintain a routine of learning something. You might want to read the newspaper on a daily basis, listen to tapes or the radio, or even just listen to people.

In addition to traditional reading and listening, there are numerous other ways to engage in continuous learning. Online courses, webinars, and podcasts offer a wealth of knowledge on a variety of topics. Many of these resources are free or low-cost, making them accessible to anyone with an internet connection.

Attending workshops, seminars, and conferences is another excellent way to learn and stay motivated. These events provide opportunities to hear from experts in your field, network with like-minded individuals, and gain new insights and perspectives.

Joining a book club or study group can also be a great way to encourage continuous learning. These groups provide a structured environment for discussing ideas, asking questions, and deepening your understanding of a subject.

Keeping a learning journal is a helpful tool for tracking your progress and reflecting on what you have learned. Writing down your thoughts and insights can reinforce your learning and help you apply it to your life.

Setting specific learning goals can help you stay focused and motivated. Whether it is mastering a new skill, exploring a new subject, or reading a certain number of books each year, having clear objectives can guide your learning efforts.

Finally, embracing a growth mindset is crucial for continuous learning. This means believing that your abilities and intelligence can be developed through dedication and hard work. With a growth mindset, you are more likely to embrace challenges, persist in the face of setbacks, and see effort as the path to mastery.

By incorporating continuous learning into your daily routine, you can keep your mind active, stay motivated, and open yourself up to new possibilities and opportunities. Whether through reading, listening, participating in educational events, or setting learning goals, there are countless ways to engage in lifelong learning and personal growth.

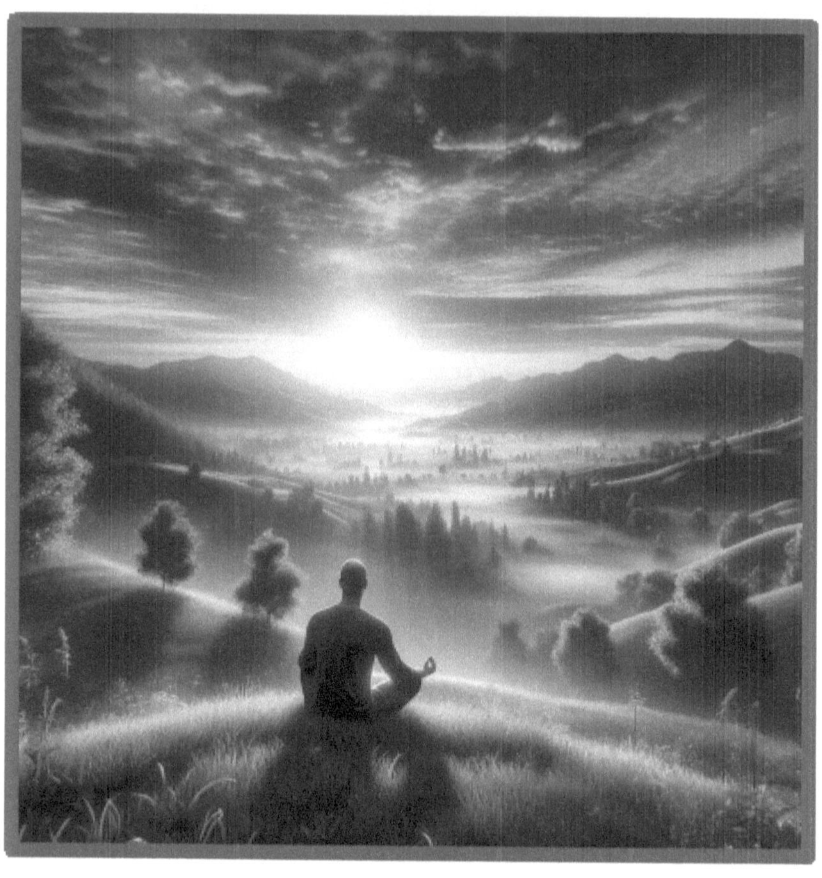

Chapter 5 – The Power of Positive Thinking

Positive thinking is key to your entire lifestyle. If you want to achieve a goal, you must be positive. Positive thinking can be achieved in so many ways and it is what will help you become motivated to do things in your life. If you are negative about achieving a goal, you will procrastinate and not want to work toward the goal. There are many ways you can maintain a positive attitude.

One way to cultivate positive thinking is through affirmations. These are positive statements that you repeat to yourself, which can help to reprogram your subconscious mind and change your negative thought patterns. For example, if you are aiming to be more confident, you might repeat to yourself, "I am confident and capable in all that I do." By consistently affirming your positive qualities, you can start to believe in them more strongly.

Visualization is another powerful tool for positive thinking. It involves creating a mental image of yourself achieving your goals. When you visualize your success, you not only increase your motivation to work towards your goals, but you also train your brain to recognize the resources and opportunities that will help you achieve them.

Gratitude is also intricately linked to positive thinking. By focusing on what you are thankful for, you shift your attention away from negative thoughts and emotions. Keeping a gratitude journal and writing down a few things you are grateful for each day can be a simple yet effective way to cultivate a positive mindset.

Surrounding yourself with positive influences is another important aspect of maintaining a positive attitude. This includes choosing to spend time with people who uplift and inspire you, as well as consuming media that is encouraging and empowering. When you are surrounded by positivity, it becomes easier to maintain a positive outlook on life.

Positive thinking is not just about being optimistic in the face of challenges; it is also about approaching problems with a constructive attitude. Instead of dwelling on the difficulties, focus on finding solutions and learning from the experience. This proactive approach can help you overcome obstacles more effectively.

It is important to recognize that positive thinking does not mean ignoring reality or pretending that everything is perfect. It is about acknowledging the challenges but choosing to focus on the opportunities and solutions. This balanced perspective can help you navigate life's ups and downs with resilience and grace.

Incorporating mindfulness and meditation into your routine can also support positive thinking. These practices help you stay present and reduce stress, which can make it easier to maintain a positive outlook. Even just a few minutes of mindfulness or meditation each day can make a significant difference in your overall mindset.

Finally, setting realistic goals and celebrating your achievements can reinforce positive thinking. When you set achievable goals and recognize your progress, you build confidence and a sense of accomplishment. This positive reinforcement encourages you to continue striving for success.

By integrating these strategies into your life, you can harness the power of positive thinking to enhance your motivation, resilience, and overall well-being. Remember, your thoughts have a profound impact on your actions and outcomes, so choose to focus on the positive and watch as it transforms your life.

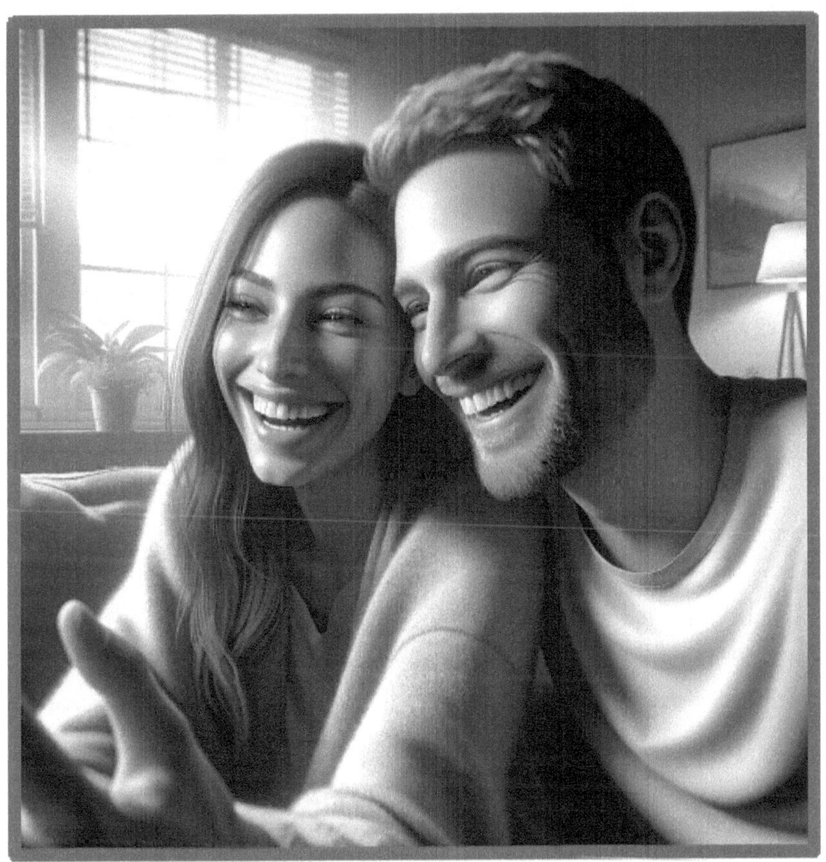

Focus on the Important Things

It is quite common for people to focus their energy on things that are not important. When your emotional energy is spent on things that are not important, it can be very draining. The first thing you need to do is to be noticeably clear about the things in your life that are important to you. Create a mission and a vision for your life and your goals. These things are important to you. This way, when you become upset about something, you can take a step back when you get upset and decide if it really is worth the energy or not. In most cases, you will find that you are wasting energy and getting upset about certain circumstances and things that you should not. This can be unhealthy and is unbelievably bad. When you are clear about the important things, you will maintain a positive attitude and you will not get upset as much.

To focus on the important things, it is essential to prioritize your tasks and responsibilities. Determine what is enormously important and what is urgent. Often, we confuse the two and end up spending time on urgent tasks that are not necessarily important in the long run. By distinguishing between the two, you can allocate your time and energy more effectively.

Another strategy is to set clear goals and objectives. When you have a clear understanding of what you want to achieve, it becomes easier to focus on the activities that will help you reach your goals. Break down your goals into smaller, manageable tasks and focus on completing them one at a time.

It is also important to learn to say no. Many people struggle with this because they do not want to disappoint others or miss opportunities. However, saying yes to everything can lead to overcommitment and distract you from your priorities. Be selective about the commitments you take on and ensure they align with your important goals.

Practicing mindfulness and being present in the moment can also help you focus on the important things. When you are fully engaged in the present, you are less likely to be distracted by non-essential tasks or worries about the future. Mindfulness techniques, such as meditation or deep breathing, can help you cultivate this sense of presence.

Simplifying your life can also contribute to focusing on what is important. This can mean decluttering your physical space, streamlining your daily routine, or eliminating unnecessary activities. By reducing the number of distractions and commitments in your life, you can free up more time and energy for the things that truly matter.

Finally, regularly review and reassess your priorities. What is important to you can change over time, so it is essential to periodically reflect on your goals and values. This will help you stay aligned with your priorities and make adjustments as needed.

By focusing on the important things, you can lead a more fulfilling and purposeful life. You will be able to invest your time and energy in activities that align with your values and goals, leading to greater satisfaction and success. Remember, it is not about doing more, but rather about doing what matters most.

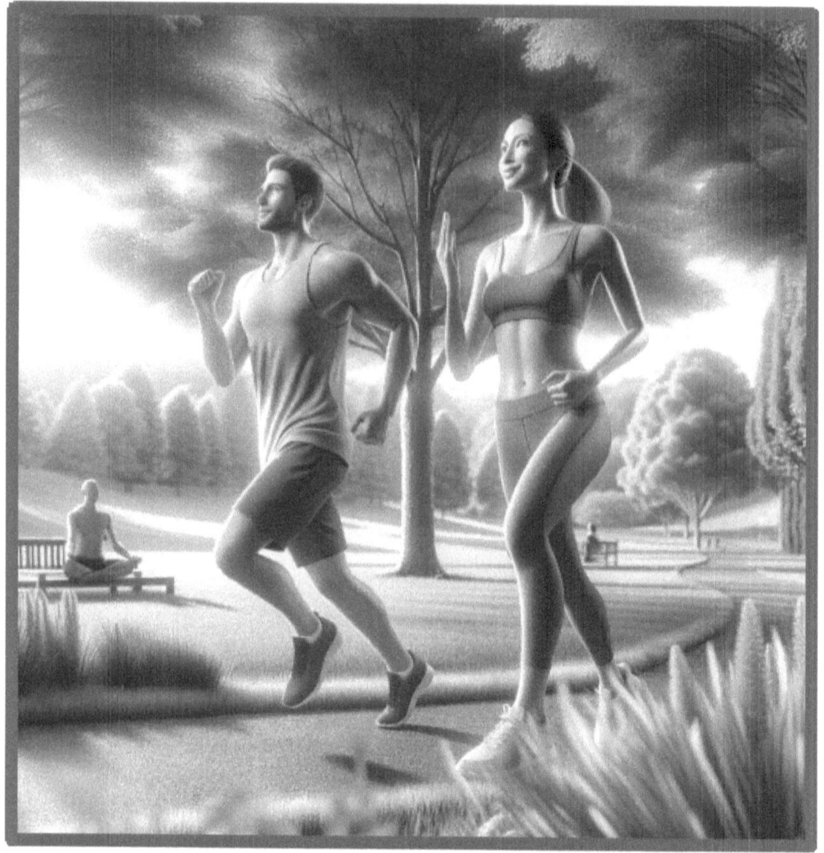

Maintain Good Health

Motivation also means you must be a healthy person. You cannot have a positive attitude when you do not take care of your body. There are three primary things you need to do in order to create a healthy body. These things include eating right, sleep, and getting plenty of exercise.

Your diet can have a lot to do with the way you feel on a daily basis. A balanced diet can make you feel good every day and positive. If you drink too much soda, you might develop a caffeine addiction which causes headaches. This can not only cause a bad attitude because you have a headache, but you also will not be motivated to do anything either.

Eating a balanced and healthy diet means cutting out the fatty foods, the sugars, alcohol, and other things that get you down. A balanced diet can help you lose weight too. Being overweight can be a factor that causes you to be unhappy with yourself and have a negative attitude. The best diet is one full of fruits, vegetables, fish and chicken, and a lot of water. Watch your portion sizes too. If you are consuming the right foods, you might just need to cut down on the sizes of portions you eat.

Exercise is also important to have a good attitude. Everyone should exercise on a daily basis. You should take at least 15 minutes every day to exercise. You do not have to do aerobics or something too strenuous. Walking is the best thing you can do for your body. A brisk 15-minute walk every day will make you feel great and completely change your attitude. This will also make you motivated and create a positive attitude about the directions you can go in your life.

If you are someone who is restricted to a desk for a large portion of your day and you do not think you have time to exercise, that is just an excuse. There are desk exercises you can do while you are sitting at your desk. During your lunch hour, you might choose to walk around the exterior of the building or even in the hallways of the interior of the building too. The stairs at your work could create an excellent workout also.

In addition to these core elements, staying hydrated is crucial for maintaining good health. Drinking plenty of water throughout the day can help keep your body functioning properly and can improve your overall mood and energy levels.

Getting enough sleep is another essential aspect of good health. Aim for 7-9 hours of quality sleep each night to help your body recover and recharge. Lack of sleep can lead to fatigue, irritability, and a lack of motivation.

Managing stress is also important for maintaining good health. Practice stress-reduction techniques such as deep breathing, meditation, or yoga to help keep your stress levels in check. A calm and relaxed mind is more conducive to motivation and positive thinking.

Regular check-ups with your healthcare provider are important to ensure that you are in good health and to address any potential health issues early on. Preventive care is key to maintaining long-term health and well-being.

Lastly, remember that maintaining good health is a continuous process. It requires making conscious choices every day to support your physical and mental well-being. By prioritizing your health, you are laying the foundation for a more motivated and fulfilling life.

In conclusion, maintaining good health is essential for sustaining motivation and a positive attitude. By focusing on a balanced diet, regular exercise, adequate sleep, hydration, stress management, and preventive care, you can support your overall well-being and enhance your ability to achieve your goals.

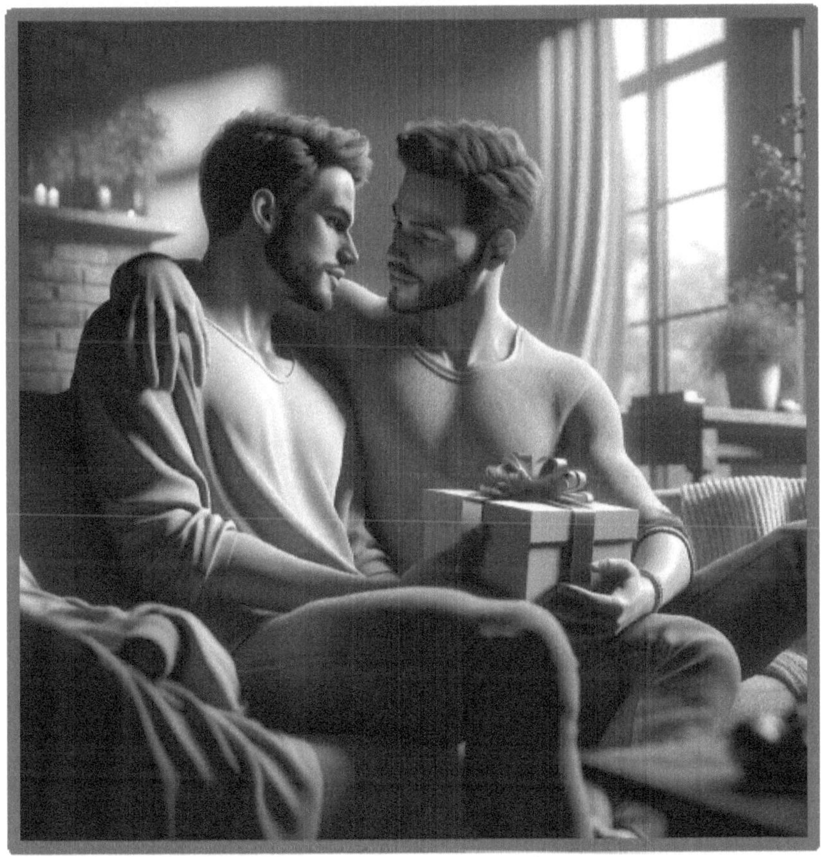

Share

Another thing you can do to create a positive attitude is to give. Giving means not only gifts but your time, attention, and energy. You might give yourself by spending time with people who need it. Spend time with a friend in the hospital or do something to boost someone's attitude. One of the best ways to boost your attitude and feel great is by giving to people.

You might give gifts, but you do not have to spend money. It is really simple to take five minutes out of your day to do something nice for someone else. In addition, it is common you will run across situations that are the perfect opportunity for you to step in and help them out. So many times, people are stuck on the side of the road with a broken-down vehicle, and no one stops to help them like they used to. People just drive by and assume the person has a cell phone. Help might mean giving someone the fifty cents they are short at the checkout or assisting the neighbor with building a fence.

Volunteering is another excellent way to give back and create a positive attitude. By dedicating your time and skills to a cause you care about, you can make a meaningful difference in the lives of others. Whether it is helping out at a local food bank, mentoring a young person, or participating in community clean-up events, volunteering can provide a sense of purpose and fulfillment.

In addition to giving to others, it is important to give to yourself as well. This means taking care of your own needs and being available for activities that bring you joy and relaxation. By nurturing your own well-being, you will be better equipped to give to others with a genuine and positive attitude.

Another aspect of giving is practicing kindness and compassion in your daily interactions. Small acts of kindness, such as holding the door open for someone, offering a compliment, or simply smiling at a stranger, can have a ripple effect and contribute to a more positive and connected community.

It is also important to be generous with your forgiveness. Holding onto grudges and resentment can weigh you down and prevent you from experiencing true happiness. By forgiving others and letting go of past hurts, you open yourself up to more positive experiences and relationships.

Giving can also extend to sharing your knowledge and expertise. Whether it is teaching a skill, offering advice, or sharing valuable insights, imparting your wisdom to others can be incredibly rewarding and help foster a culture of learning and growth.

Finally, remember that giving is not just about what you do for others, but also about the attitude with which you do it. Giving with a genuine and joyful heart, without expecting anything in return, is the true essence of generosity. By embracing the power of giving, you can create a more positive attitude for yourself and spread happiness and kindness to those around you.

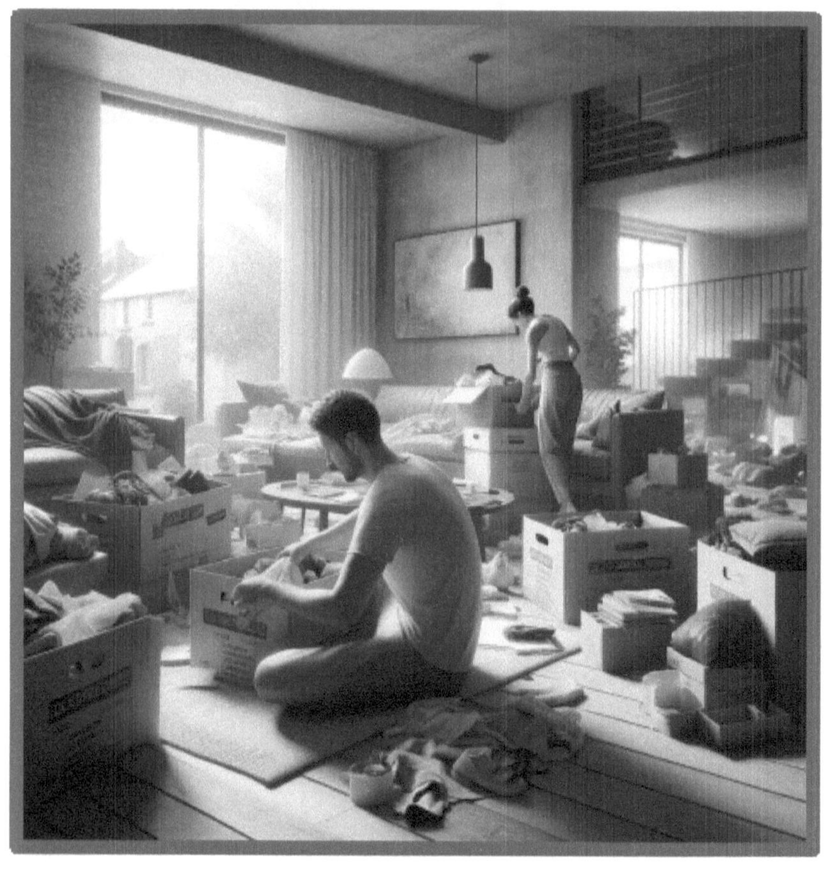

Get Rid of Unnecessary Items

If your home is cluttered with things, you do not need or that are just taking up space, you might consider giving them away. The old saying that 'someone else's junk is another's treasure' really does ring true. You might be so focused on possessions and the things that you own that you really do not enjoy life as you should. Maybe you grew up with nothing, which is why possessions are so important to you. One of the best ways to feel good about yourself and give yourself an immediate boost is to give. When you realize those possessions, you own and realize they really are not that important to you, giving them away is an excellent boost. You will feel very great about yourself.

Decluttering your home can have a significant impact on your mental and emotional well-being. By getting rid of items that no longer serve a purpose in your life, you create a more peaceful and organized living environment. This can lead to reduced stress levels, improved focus, and a greater sense of calm.

When deciding what to give away, consider items that you have not used in a long time, things that no longer fit your lifestyle or interests, and duplicates of items you already have. By letting go of these things, you not only free up physical space but also make room for new experiences and opportunities.

Donating items to charity is a wonderful way to give back to your community and help those in need. Many organizations accept a variety of items, including clothing, household goods, and furniture. By donating, you can provide essential items to people who may not be able to afford them otherwise.

In addition to physical items, consider giving your time and talents. Volunteering at a local charity, offering your skills to help a friend or neighbor, or simply being there for someone in need can be incredibly rewarding. The act of giving your time and energy can be just as fulfilling as giving away material possessions.

It is important to remember that giving should come from a place of genuine desire to help and not from a sense of obligation or expectation of something in return. When you give freely and with an open heart, the positive impact on both the giver and the receiver is immeasurable.

Giving can also be a way to practice gratitude and mindfulness. By focusing on what you can give rather than what you lack, you cultivate a mindset of abundance and appreciation. This shift in perspective can lead to increased happiness and satisfaction in life.

As you declutter and give away items, take the time to reflect on the reasons behind your attachment to material possessions.

Understanding the emotional or psychological factors that drive your behavior can lead to deeper self-awareness and personal growth.

Finally, consider the environmental benefits of giving away items rather than throwing them away. By repurposing or recycling items, you contribute to a more sustainable and eco-friendlier world. This act of kindness extends beyond the immediate recipients of your donations and has a positive impact on the planet as a whole.

In conclusion, giving away possessions that no longer serve you can be a powerful way to declutter your home, support your community, and boost your own well-being. By focusing on what truly matters and letting go of the rest, you can live a more meaningful and fulfilling life.

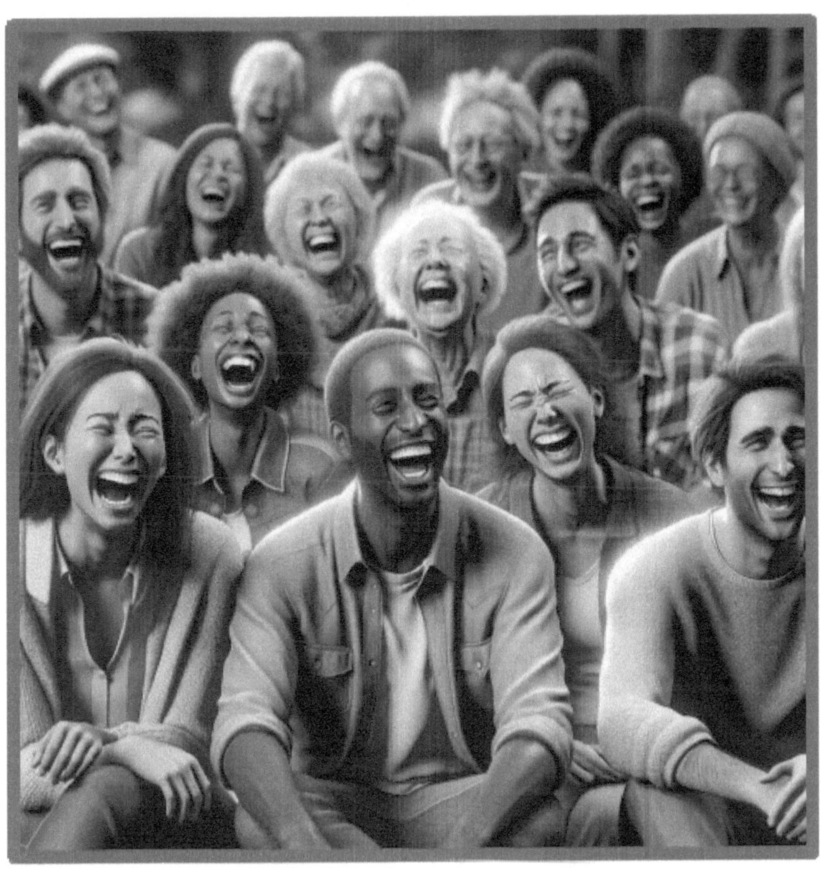

Look at the Funny Side

Life is funny. When you see the funny side of life and the humor in things, you will have an excellent attitude. You will find the people who have the best attitude often have the best sense of humor. When you have a good sense of humor, you will feel great about life and be positive too. A positive mind is someone who sees the good in life and in even the little things. This can also help you create motivation so you can move forward and achieve the goals you will set.

If you are someone who tends to be serious about just about everything, you might want to take a step back and see the funny side of life. Being too serious can only cause stress and worry. When you are stressed and worried, you are also focusing on negative things. Focus on the funny and the positive. In most cases, you might be able to find something funny about most things.

Laughter is often called the best medicine for a good reason. It has numerous health benefits, including reducing stress, boosting your immune system, and even relieving pain. By incorporating more humor into your life, you can improve your physical and mental well-being.

One way to see the funny side of life is to surround yourself with people who have a good sense of humor. Spend time with friends and family who make you laugh and feel good. Their positive energy can be contagious and help you adopt a more lighthearted perspective.

Watching comedies, reading humorous books, or listening to funny podcasts are also great ways to inject humor into your life. These forms of entertainment can provide a much-needed escape from the seriousness of everyday life and remind you to laugh at the absurdities.

Practicing self-deprecation can also be a healthy way to see the funny side of life. Being able to laugh at yourself shows a sense of confidence and can help you navigate difficult situations with grace. It is important, however, to strike a balance and not be overly self-critical.

Learning to find humor in challenging situations can also be a valuable coping mechanism. When faced with adversity, try to find a silver lining or a humorous angle. This can help you maintain a positive outlook and resilience in the face of obstacles.

It is also important to be mindful of the type of humor you engage in. While humor can be a powerful tool for positivity, it should never be at the expense of others. Practice kindness and empathy in your humor to ensure that it uplifts rather than hurts.

Finally, remember that humor is subjective. What one person finds funny, another may not. Be open to different types of humor and do not be afraid to explore new comedic styles. By broadening your sense of humor, you can enrich your life and bring more joy into your daily experiences.

In conclusion, looking at the funny side of life can have a profound impact on your attitude and overall well-being. By embracing humor, surrounding yourself with positive influences, and finding laughter in the midst of challenges, you can cultivate a more joyful and resilient outlook on life.

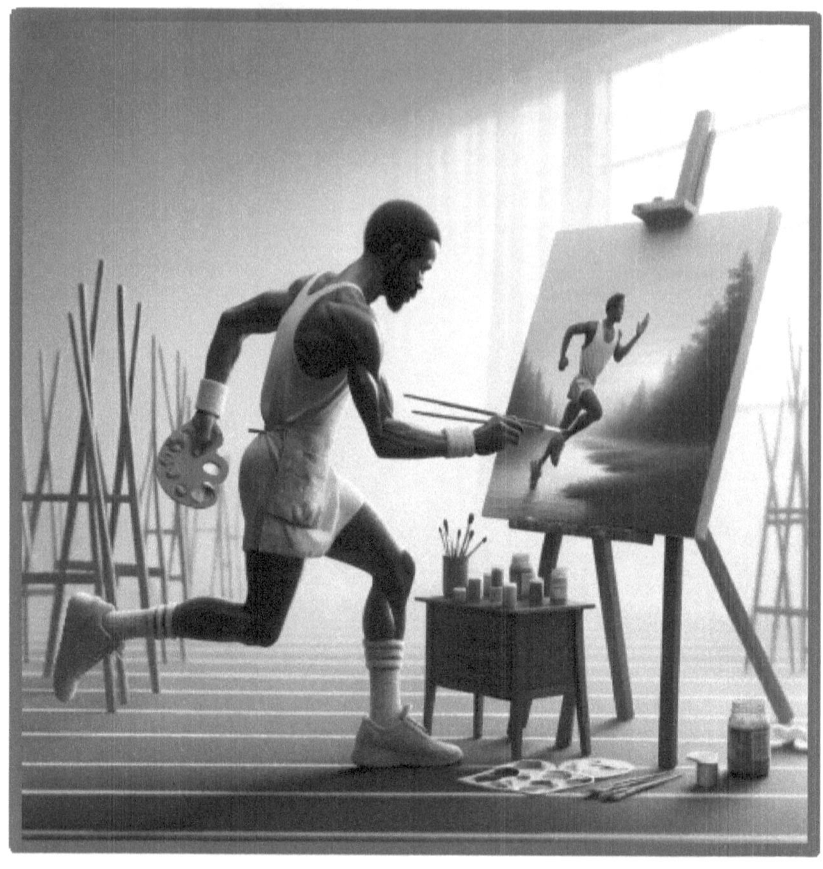

Focus on Your Strengths

Everyone has strengths and is good at something. You might be one of the millions of people who are working a job that does you no justice. You might have qualifications far beyond what you are doing every day. This is a goal you can set for yourself to use your strengths. However, on a daily basis, you can practice the things you enjoy and the things at which you are good. If you do not have the time to do these things every day, you should put time aside to do these things at least three times a week or even throughout the weekend.

When you focus on things you are good at, it makes you feel good. You should have a hobby if you are unable to do these things while you are working every day. If you love arts and crafts or writing, you should spend the time doing these things. This can help you become positive. When you focus on strengths and things you enjoy, you will also become motivated to achieve goals focused on these things. This might include entering a contest or applying for a job.

The best thing you can do for yourself is to play on your strengths. Think about the things that you enjoy doing. Think about the things you are good at. You know you are good at something. You should think about these things and begin to focus on them. Set time aside for yourself to enjoy these things. Do not think of something you are good at that you despise. Be sure you focus on something that makes you feel good. If you are not good at this task, it is still okay. You can be the worst painter, but if it makes you feel good and positive, then you should continue. Pay no attention to any negativity that comes your way during this time also.

One last point, when you choose things to do that make you feel good about yourself, be sure these things are healthy for you. If you feel great when you drink wine because you forget about the bad, it could create a problem. Choose a skill or something positive for you that makes you feel good.

By focusing on your strengths, you can build self-confidence and self-esteem. When you recognize and celebrate your abilities, you reinforce a positive self-image. This can lead to a virtuous cycle where success in one area of your life fuels motivation and confidence in other areas.

It is also important to seek feedback from others about your strengths. Sometimes, others can see talents and abilities in you that you might not recognize yourself. This feedback can provide valuable insights and help you identify areas where you can further develop your strengths.

In addition to focusing on your strengths, it is beneficial to work on improving your weaknesses. However, this should not be at the expense of neglecting your strengths. Striking a balance between developing your strengths and addressing your weaknesses is key to personal and professional growth.

Setting goals that align with your strengths can also help you stay motivated and engaged. When you set goals that play to your strengths, you are more likely to enjoy the process of working towards them and achieving success.

Remember that your strengths can evolve over time. As you gain new experiences and learn new skills, your strengths may change. Regularly reflecting on your strengths and how they align with your goals and values can help you stay focused and adapt to changes in your life.

In conclusion, focusing on your strengths is a powerful way to enhance your well-being and achieve success. By recognizing and leveraging your unique talents and abilities, you can create a fulfilling life that brings you joy and satisfaction. Remember to celebrate your strengths, seek feedback, set goals that align with your strengths, and be open to growth and change.

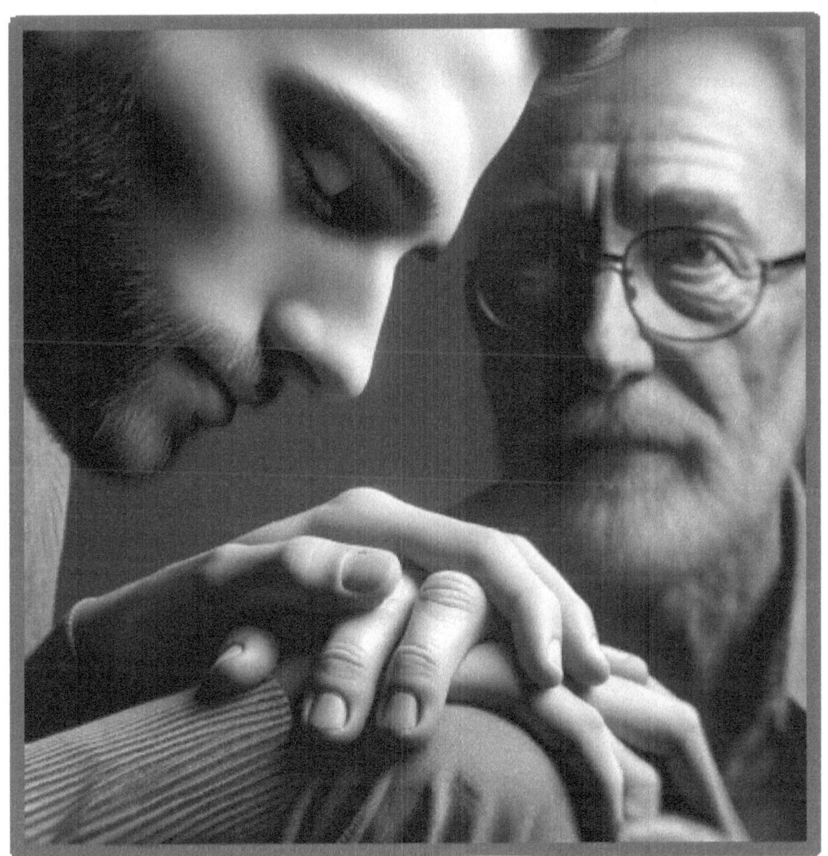

Building buffers

Buffers are important in your life. As you go through life, you will find there are certain circumstances that you have absolutely no control of. Most things in life are out of your control. You should not try to control anyone or have too much control over the things that happen in your life. Your positive attitude will help you manage your life and the things you do. You need to create buffers, so you accept the fact that you do not have control over the circumstance.

When you create buffers, you might choose to talk to friends to work you through certain circumstances. You might choose to talk to a counselor or a therapist to make it through a hard time. Many people practice meditation to help them accept they do not have control over the realities faced throughout the days. You might want to build an external support system so when the bad does strike, you have people to talk you through the hard times.

Building buffers also means setting healthy boundaries in your relationships and personal life. By establishing clear boundaries, you protect your mental and emotional well-being from being overwhelmed by external pressures or demands. This can include saying no to additional responsibilities when you are already stretched thin or limiting your exposure to negative influences.

Another way to build buffers is to practice self-care regularly. This can include activities such as exercise, getting enough sleep, eating a balanced diet, and engaging in hobbies or activities that bring you joy. By taking care of your physical and mental health, you strengthen your resilience and ability to cope with life's challenges.

Financial buffers are also important for peace of mind. Setting aside savings for emergencies or unexpected expenses can provide a sense of security and reduce stress in times of financial uncertainty.

Mindfulness and stress reduction techniques can also serve as buffers. Techniques such as deep breathing, progressive muscle relaxation, or guided imagery can help you stay centered and calm in the face of adversity.

Developing a growth mindset can also be a buffer against life's challenges. By viewing obstacles as opportunities for growth and learning, you can maintain a positive outlook and adapt more easily to change.

Cultivating a strong support network is another key aspect of building buffers. Having a circle of friends, family, or colleagues who offer emotional support and understanding can make a significant difference in how you navigate difficult situations.

It is also important to recognize when you need to seek professional help. If you are struggling to cope with stress, anxiety, depression, or other mental health issues, reaching out to a mental health professional can provide the guidance and support you need to build effective buffers.

In conclusion, building buffers in your life involves a combination of self-care, setting boundaries, financial planning, stress reduction techniques, cultivating a positive mindset, and seeking support when needed. By proactively creating these protective measures, you can better navigate the uncertainties of life and maintain your well-being in the face of challenges.

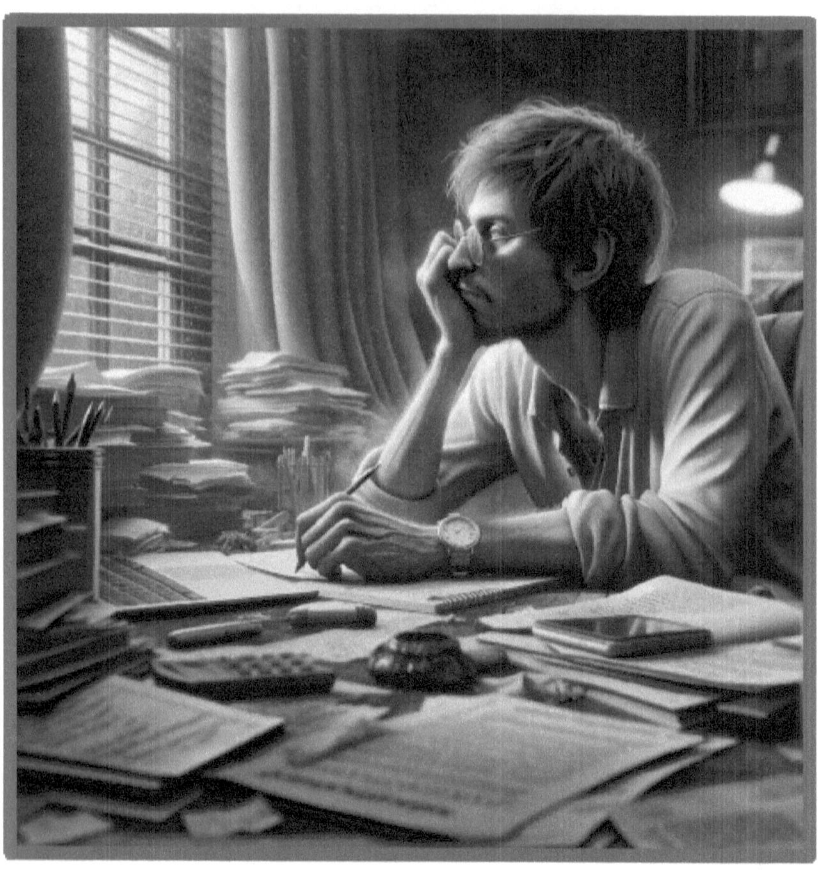

Chapter 6 – Procrastination

Procrastination can be the reason you do not make it through many tasks throughout the day. You might find you get drawn into a television show or playing on the Internet. When you look at the clock, the day has gone by, and you have not completed any of your work. This lack of productivity will cause you to be very unmotivated.

Procrastination can be damaging. The effects can also be damaging if your procrastination causes problems with your work life, personal life, and more. Putting things off is a serious problem for many people, and you need to get the ball rolling.

Many people are very aware they procrastinate but they cannot get out of the funk they are stuck in. You can. It is common to sit around and think about how things could be or how things will be. You might have a project you need to complete and sit around and think about doing the project but never get started with it. You might meet deadlines at the last minute. This does not make anyone feel good about themselves.

If your motivation is lacking on a project, you might consider changing the focus to something else that needs to get done. If you have a paper due and you cannot get focused do not sit in front of the computer and play. Find something else around the house to get done and then go back to get the paper done. Starting another task may give you the momentum you need to get rolling with the project you need to get done.

Procrastination can be very damaging. You might be aware or unaware of the procrastination you suffer with. However, you need to pay attention to the time you spend sitting around doing nothing. When you can beat procrastination and you become entirely productive you will be incredibly positive about life. You will also be motivated to take on new projects too because you will be spending less time sitting around.

One effective strategy to combat procrastination is to break down large tasks into smaller, more manageable steps. This can make the task feel less overwhelming and more achievable. Setting deadlines for each step can also help keep you on track.

Using a planner or a to-do list can help you organize your tasks and prioritize them based on urgency and importance. This can provide a clear roadmap for what needs to be done and help you stay focused.

Another useful technique is the Pomodoro Technique, which involves working for a set period (usually 25 minutes), followed by a short break. This can help improve concentration and productivity by providing a structured approach to work.

It is also important to identify and address any underlying reasons for procrastination. This could include fear of failure, perfectionism, or lack of interest in the task. Understanding the root cause can help you develop strategies to overcome these obstacles.

Creating a conducive work environment can also make a big difference. Minimize distractions, such as turning off notifications on your phone or computer, and ensure you have all the necessary tools and resources at hand.

Rewarding yourself for completing tasks can also be a great motivator. Treat yourself to something you enjoy, whether it is a small treat, a break to do something you love, or simply acknowledging your progress.

Finally, be kind to yourself. Procrastination is a common issue, and it is important to recognize that progress takes time. Celebrate your successes, no matter how small, and remember that every step forward is a step in the right direction.

In conclusion, overcoming procrastination requires a combination of strategies, including breaking tasks into smaller steps, using planning tools, addressing underlying issues, creating a productive work environment, and rewarding yourself for progress. By taking these steps, you can boost your productivity, enhance your motivation, and achieve your goals more effectively.

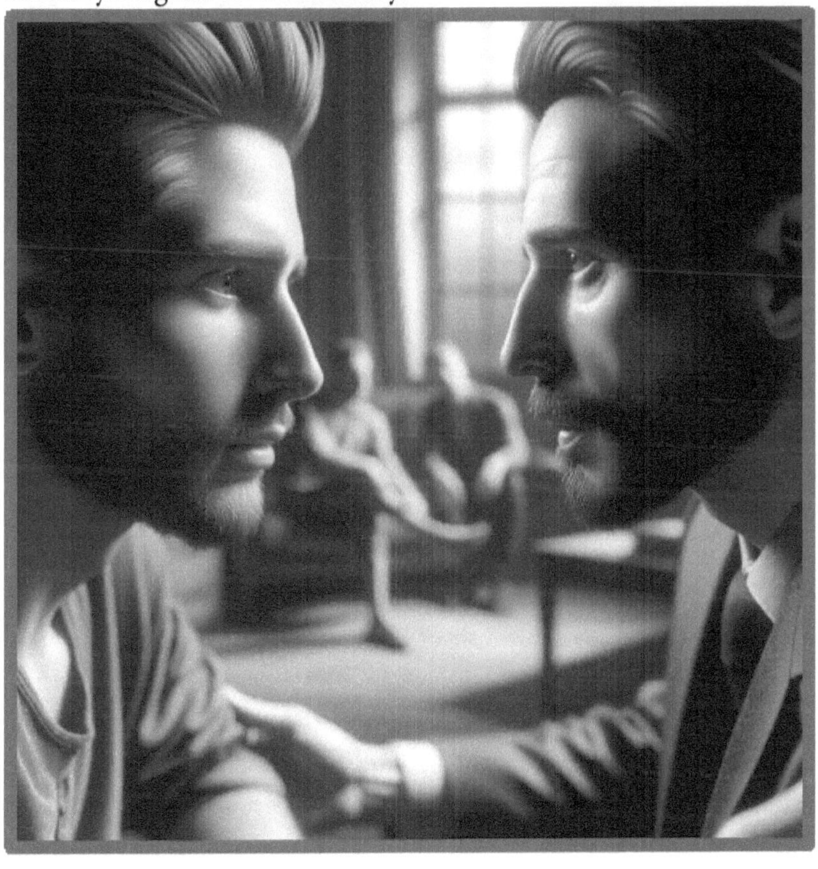

Chapter 7 – Knowing Yourself

One of the ways you can work on a daily basis to motivate yourself is to get to know yourself. You need to focus on yourself and think about the things that make you feel good and the things that make you feel bad.

Writing is an extremely healthy way to get to know you. You might want to try writing in a journal or making use of lists. Lists can be extremely helpful for becoming positive and getting to know you. First, make a list of the things that you feel good about. These might be from the first cup of coffee in the morning, a fresh pair of socks, or achieving a big goal.

Write a list of all of the things that you enjoy doing and the things that you like. This list can help you create a positive atmosphere by surrounding yourself around positive things in your life. This list will also help you create better and more positive days. You will feel motivated to design a life full of the positive things that make you happy.

You should also write about the things that are negative in your life and the things that bother you. This list should include everything that might cause you to feel negative about days or events in your life. They might impact you in some way. You might have a chair in your living room you absolutely hate. Put it on your list of things to do to get rid of it immediately.

Once you have the negative list put together, you need to begin making sure these items and behaviors are taken out of your life. Think of the ways you can design your days around only the positive things without the negativity.

When you get to know yourself, it is the best thing you can do. It is important to understand the things that make you feel positive and the things that bring negative emotions to you. The better you can design your life in a positive fashion, you will be entirely motivated to live it thoroughly.

In addition to writing, engaging in self-reflection is another way to get to know yourself better. Take time to contemplate your values, beliefs, and priorities. Understanding what truly matters to you can guide your decisions and actions, leading to a more fulfilling life.

Exploring your interests and trying new things can also help you discover more about yourself. Whether it is taking up a new hobby, learning a new skill, or traveling to new places, these experiences can reveal aspects of your personality and preferences that you may not have been aware of.

Setting aside time for solitude can be beneficial for self-discovery. In our busy lives, it is easy to get caught up in the noise and distractions of the world. By spending time alone, you can tune into your inner thoughts and feelings without external influences.

Seeking feedback from others can provide valuable insights into your character and behavior. Sometimes, friends, family, and colleagues can offer perspectives that you might not have considered. However, it is important to discern constructive feedback from criticism and to use it as a tool for growth.

Practicing mindfulness and being present in the moment can help you become more attuned to your emotions and reactions. This awareness can be instrumental in understanding yourself and managing your responses to different situations.

Embracing your uniqueness and accepting yourself as you are a key aspect of knowing yourself. Celebrate your strengths and acknowledge your weaknesses without judgment. Self-acceptance is a crucial step towards self-improvement and personal growth.

In conclusion, knowing yourself is a continuous journey that involves introspection, exploration, and self-acceptance. By dedicating time to understand what makes you tick, you can create a life that aligns with your true self and enhances your motivation to pursue your goals and dreams.

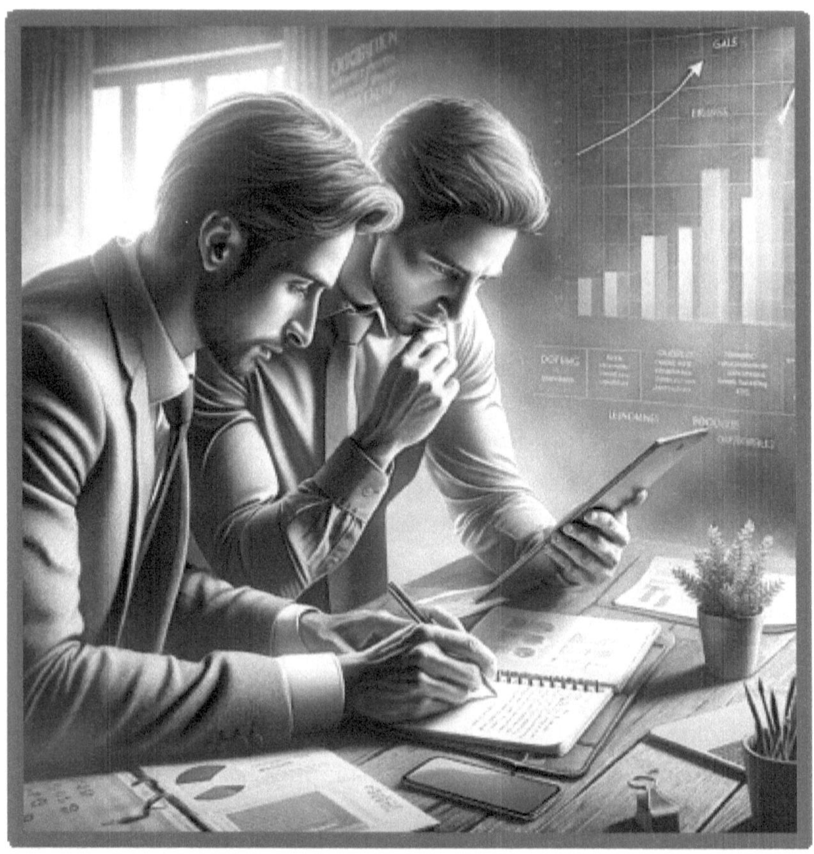

Chapter 8 – Goal Setting and Tracking Progress

Goal setting is the most important thing. If you do not have any goals in life, you must be pretty bored. Some people sit around every day and say they are content with going back and forth to work at the same job every single day, year after year. You see nothing happen and you can always guess where they will be because they never do anything out of their routine. You might be one of these people.

Setting goals helps you grow. It makes you feel good to set goals and work toward making them happen. Goal setting is healthy for your body and healthy for your mind. One of the things to consider when it comes to setting goals is that you do not want to sit around and talk about the goals you have. This will do you nothing but be discouraging.

When you set goals, they have to be realistic and reachable, or you will be discouraged. Always set goals that you really can reach, and you see a way to meet them. It is important to write down the steps it will take to accomplish the goal. Decide how long it will take you to accomplish each task. This might be in days or weeks. Once you do this you will need to set a date that you will begin working toward the goal. Then you can set the project up on a calendar and write down where you should be with each task.

As you begin a project or a completion of a goal you must track the progress. As you meet certain milestones you need to treat yourself to something special because you are one step closer to doing something you feel is important. If you are running behind, you might need to pick it up a step or extend out the deadline. Be sure that you are only running behind because you underestimated, and you are really working according to your task.

Goal setting is especially important. When you set goals and lay them out with times and milestones you will be more motivated to complete them. As you reach certain milestones you will be motivated more than ever to reach the end of the project. This is an incredibly positive way to work on projects, especially if you have a hard time completing them.

In addition to setting realistic goals, it is important to make them specific and measurable. Instead of setting a vague goal like "I want to be healthier," set a specific goal like "I want to exercise for 30 minutes, five days a week." This makes it easier to track your progress and know when you have achieved your goal.

It is also helpful to break down larger goals into smaller, more manageable tasks. This can make the goal seem less daunting and give you a clear path to follow. Celebrating small victories along the way can keep you motivated and focused on the end goal.

Another key aspect of goal setting is flexibility. Life is unpredictable, and sometimes circumstances change that may require you to adjust your goals. Being flexible and willing to adapt your plans can help you stay on track even when faced with challenges.

Accountability is another important factor in achieving your goals. Sharing your goals with a friend, family member, or mentor can provide you with the support and encouragement you need to stay committed. They can also help hold you accountable and keep you on track.

Finally, it is important to reflect on your goals regularly. Take time to evaluate your progress, identify any obstacles you are facing, and adjust your plan as needed. This ongoing reflection can help you stay aligned with your goals and ensure you are making the progress you desire.

In conclusion, goal setting and tracking progress are essential components of personal and professional development. By setting realistic, specific, and measurable goals, breaking them down into manageable tasks, staying flexible, seeking accountability, and regularly reflecting on your progress, you can achieve your goals and create a fulfilling and successful life.

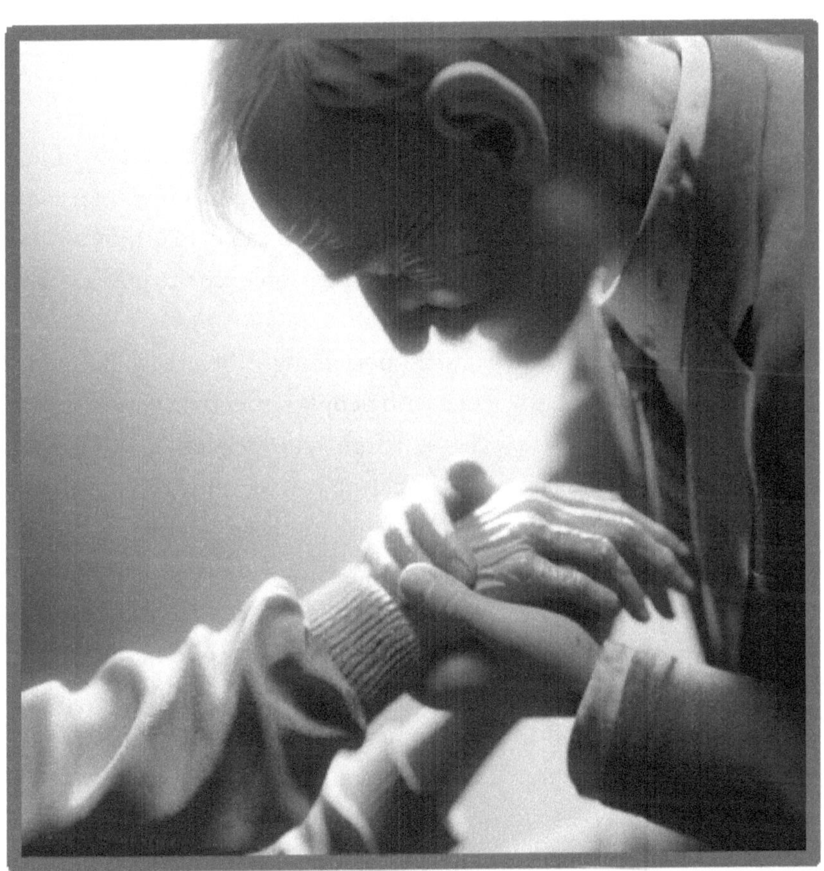

Chapter 9 – Helping Others

Helping others is especially important to make yourself feel good and feel positive about your life. When you help others, you will feel very motivated with your life. Many of the ways you can help others include sharing knowledge, visiting others, helping people see the positive, and much more.

Sharing your knowledge is a good thing. There is a difference between sharing your knowledge with people rather than your opinion. If you have something to say that is helpful and educational, it is a good thing. Be sure you are clear about offering your opinion. This will only make you feel bad later if you should hurt someone's feelings.

Knowledge sharing means you talk about the things you know. If you are educated or skilled in a specific subject maybe you can offer to teach people how to do the things you know. If you are a skilled underwater basket weaver, then share your knowledge. There are always people who are excited to learn something new. It will actually make you feel good to share your knowledge with others.

Visiting others, especially those who are lonely or in need of company, is another way to help. Whether it is spending time with an elderly neighbor, visiting someone in the hospital, or volunteering at a local shelter, your presence can make a significant difference in someone's life.

Helping people see the positive is also a valuable form of assistance. Encouraging others to focus on the good in their lives, offering a different perspective during tough times, or simply being a source of positivity can uplift those around you.

In addition to these, there are countless other ways to help others. Volunteering for community service projects, donating to charitable causes, offering a listening ear to a friend in need, or even small acts of kindness like holding the door open for someone can all contribute to making the world a better place.

Helping others can also extend to mentoring or coaching. Sharing your experiences, providing guidance, and supporting others in their personal or professional growth can be incredibly rewarding. It not only benefits the person you are helping but also enhances your own sense of purpose and fulfillment.

Acts of kindness, no matter how small, can have a ripple effect. When you help others, it often inspires them to pay it forward and help someone else in return. This creates a cycle of positivity and kindness that can spread throughout communities.

It is important to remember that helping others should come from a genuine desire to do so and not from a place of seeking recognition or reward. The true value of helping lies in the joy and satisfaction that comes from making a positive impact on someone else's life.

In conclusion, helping others is a powerful way to enrich your own life and the lives of those around you. Whether it is through sharing knowledge, offering your time, or simply being a source of positivity, every act of kindness counts. By making a commitment to help others, you can create a more compassionate, connected, and fulfilling world.

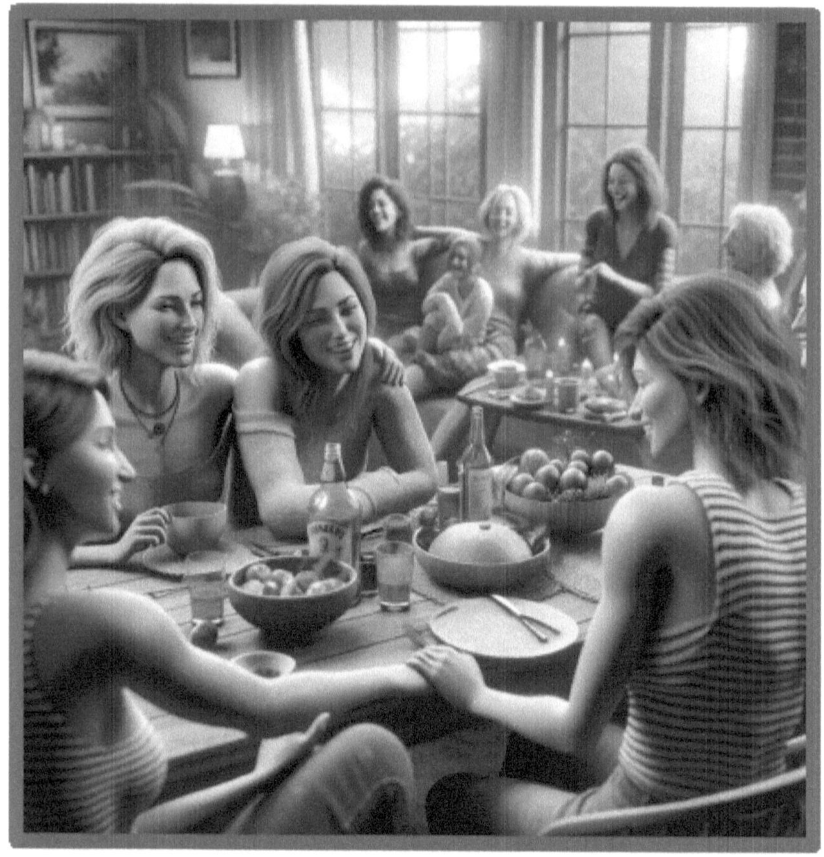

Spend Time with Friends

It is quite common for people to be negative and have a bad attitude. If you know one of these people, you do not want to spend too much time hanging out with them or seeking a positive experience, or you might find yourself becoming negative too. One of the things you can do is help these people create a more positive attitude toward life and their natural surroundings.

Some people are so negative they are extremely hard to be around. It may be frustrating. As you work toward your daily motivational techniques, you might find it hard to be around them. This is where you can make an effort to help these people. However, do not make this task so difficult that you become frustrated.

When you help negative people by spending time with them, it does not mean you are about to revolutionize their way of thinking. Your positive attitude can be contagious. When someone is down in the dumps or feeling negative, you can help them by seeing the positive side of the situation. You can help them see the good in the negative things that are happening in their lives. You can also help them realize that they have no control over the situation. The sooner someone realizes they have no control over issues in their life, they will be able to let it go and relax.

Spending time with negative friends means sharing your positive attitude. You want to share this energy but do not force it upon anyone. Do not try too hard to change someone at all.

Additionally, spending time with friends who share your positive outlook can be incredibly uplifting. Surrounding yourself with people who inspire, support, and encourage you can boost your mood and motivation. Engaging in activities that you all enjoy, having meaningful conversations, and simply enjoying each other's company can strengthen your friendships and enhance your overall well-being.

It is also important to be a good listener when spending time with friends. Sometimes, all a person needs is a sympathetic ear and someone who understands. By being there for your friends and offering support when they need it, you can help them navigate through tough times.

Remember to balance your time between helping negative friends and spending time with positive ones. While it is noble to want to help others, it is also essential to protect your own energy and well-being. Setting boundaries and knowing when to step back is crucial to maintaining your own positivity.

Creating memorable experiences with friends can also deepen your connections. Whether it is going on a trip together, trying out a new hobby, or simply having a fun night in, shared experiences can bring joy and laughter to your lives.

In conclusion, spending time with friends is a vital part of maintaining a positive outlook on life. Whether you are helping a negative friend see the brighter side of things or enjoying the company of positive friends, these relationships can provide support, joy, and a sense of belonging. By being a good friend, listener, and source of positivity, you can enhance your own life and the lives of those around you.

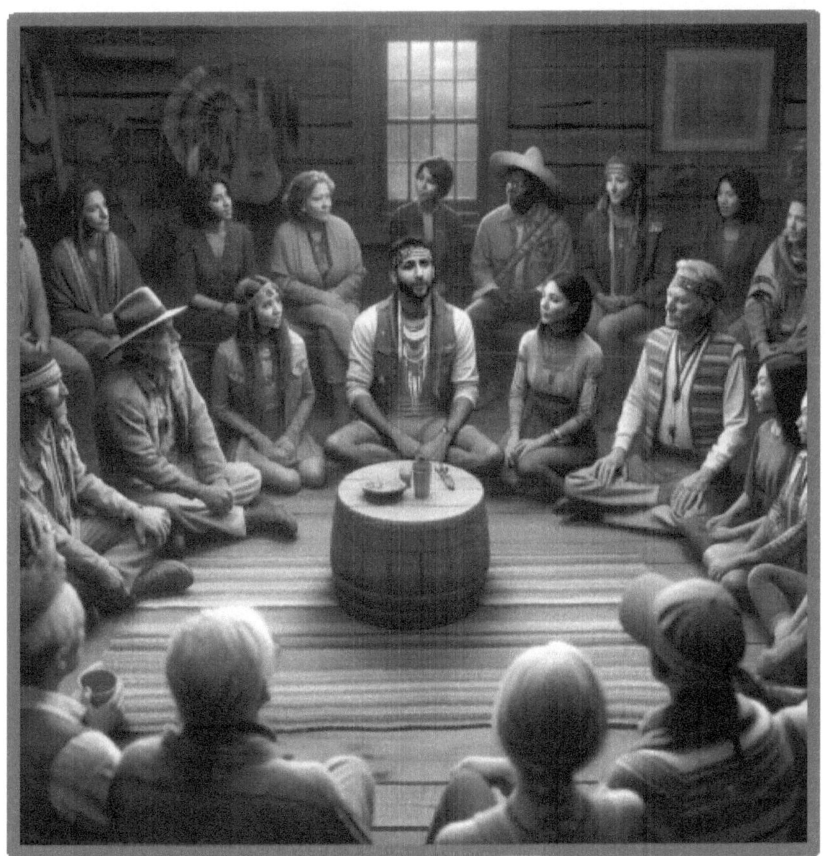

Find the Good in Other People

Everyone does have a good side, even if you do not see it immediately upon meeting them. Some people might strike you as entirely negative. Immediately upon meeting someone, the initial confrontation may be unfriendly and frustrating. Try to find the positive side in people no matter how difficult they seem to be.

When you are around negative people, they will have a negative impact on you. It is important to try and find the good in others. Everyone has good things. The better you find in others, the easier it will be to talk to them and be around them. If you are forced to be around negative people in a meeting or some other situation you cannot avoid, finding the positive will help you make it through them.

One way to find the good in others is to practice empathy. Try to put yourself in their shoes and understand their perspective. Often, people's negative behavior is a result of their own struggles or insecurities. By showing empathy, you can connect with them on a deeper level and see the good beneath the surface.

Another approach is to focus on their strengths and accomplishments. Everyone has unique talents and qualities that are worth recognizing. By acknowledging these positive aspects, you can shift your perspective and see the person in a more favorable light.

Active listening is also key to finding the good in others. When you listen attentively to what someone is saying, you can discover their values, passions, and positive traits. This can help you appreciate their uniqueness and the contributions they bring to the table.

It's also important to give people the benefit of the doubt. Sometimes, a person's negative behavior might be a result of a bad day or a misunderstanding. By giving them a chance to show their better side, you can foster a more positive relationship.

Practicing gratitude can also help you find the good in others. When you focus on the things you appreciate about a person, it becomes easier to overlook their flaws. This can lead to more harmonious interactions and a greater sense of connection.

Encouraging others to share their positive experiences or achievements can also bring out their good side. By creating an environment where people feel comfortable expressing their joys and successes, you can foster a more positive atmosphere.

In conclusion, finding the good in others is a valuable skill that can improve your relationships and overall outlook on life. By practicing empathy, focusing on strengths, listening actively, giving the benefit of the doubt, expressing gratitude, and encouraging positive sharing, you can discover the goodness in everyone you meet. This can lead to more meaningful connections and a more positive social environment.

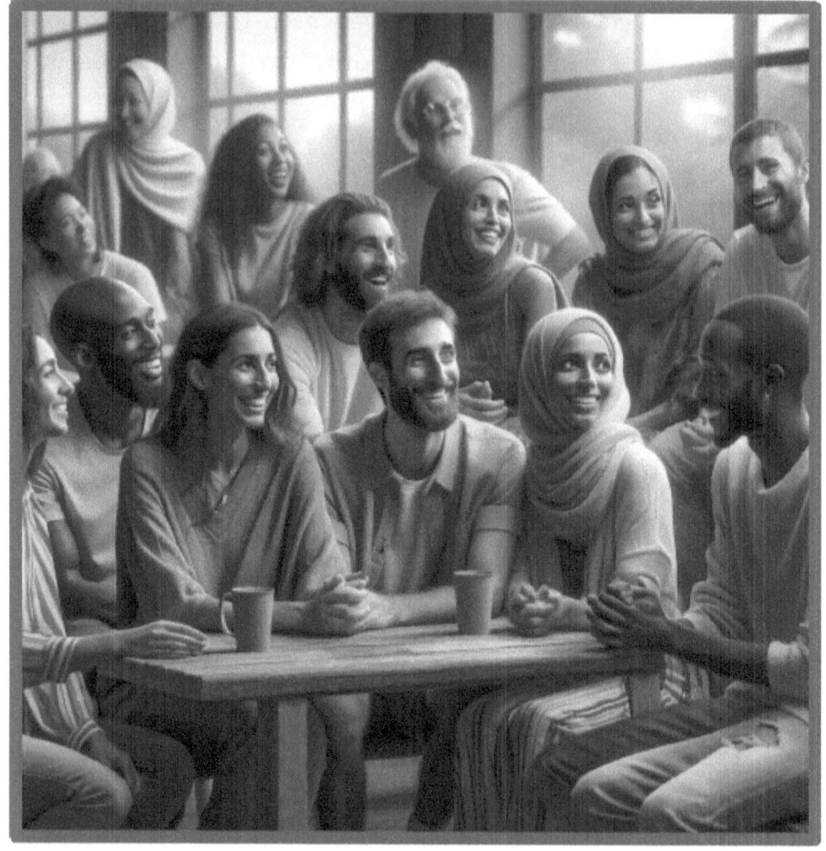

Being More Positive with Everyone

Even though you are looking for the positive aspects in negative people, you need to remain positive in everything you do. Be positive with the people you are around on a daily basis. The more positive you are to people, the more motivated you will feel too.

You do not have to suck up to anyone when you are being positive. If you are around people, you do not like, you still do not have to be negative. You can be a positive person and find the good in everything. The coffee might taste great, and you slept well. Beating the traffic is a good thing and if you did not then you had a great CD to listen to on your way to work.

It is about focusing on the little things and finding the positive in them. The more positive you find in people and the things around you, the happier you will be. You will also be more motivated to make it through every day and reach your goals.

Being more positive with everyone also means showing kindness and compassion. Small acts of kindness, such as a smile, a compliment, or offering help, can make a big difference in someone's day. These gestures not only uplift others but also enhance your own sense of well-being.

Practicing gratitude is another way to be more positive with everyone. By expressing appreciation for the people in your life and the experiences you share, you cultivate a positive outlook that is contagious.

It is also important to be an encourager. When you uplift and support others in their endeavors, you create a positive environment that fosters growth and collaboration. Encouraging others can also boost your own confidence and positivity.

Being more positive with everyone also involves being a good listener. By genuinely listening to others, you show that you value their thoughts and feelings. This can build stronger relationships and create a more positive atmosphere.

Avoiding gossip and negative talk is crucial to being more positive with everyone. Engaging in negative conversations can spread negativity and harm relationships. By steering clear of gossip, you contribute to a more positive and respectful environment.

Being adaptable and flexible can also help you be more positive with everyone. Life is unpredictable, and being able to go with the flow and maintain a positive attitude in the face of change can be inspiring to those around you.

In conclusion, being more positive with everyone involves a combination of kindness, gratitude, encouragement, active listening, avoiding negativity, and adaptability. By incorporating these practices into your interactions, you can spread positivity, build stronger relationships, and create a more uplifting environment for yourself and others.

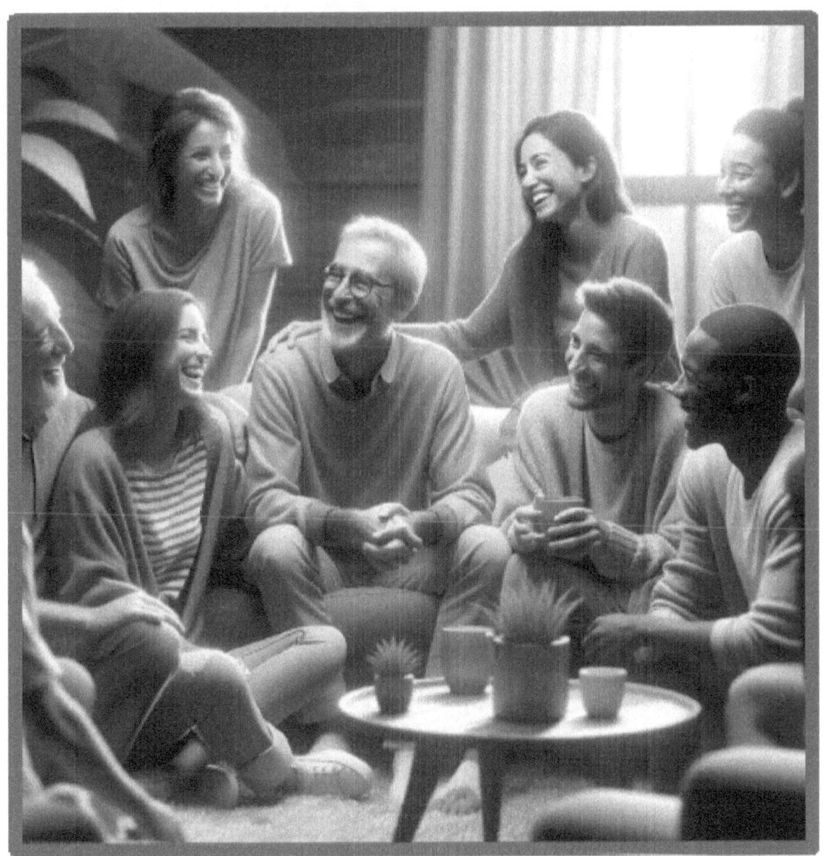

Transmit Your Positive Attitude

You might feel great and positive. Be sure to transmit your attitude to others around you and when you are indirectly talking to people too. A positive attitude is addicting, and people will enjoy spending time around you. They will feel good too. This can help you move up in the corporate world too.

When you have a positive attitude, you need to transmit it to others. This also includes when you are on the phone or on the computer. It is common for a communication disconnect to occur when you are over the phone. You might be tired or not even notice to the other person you are coming off rude. Transmit your positive attitude to others when you talk to them on the phone. This is healthy for you, and it will make the other person feel good about you.

In addition to verbal communication, your body language and non-verbal cues also play a significant role in transmitting your positive attitude. Smiling, maintaining eye contact, and using open body language can convey warmth and positivity to others.

It is also important to be mindful of the words you choose. Using positive language, focusing on solutions rather than problems, and expressing gratitude can all contribute to a positive atmosphere. Even in challenging situations, framing your words positively can make a big difference in how your message is received.

Being an active listener is another way to transmit your positive attitude. By giving others your full attention, acknowledging their feelings, and responding with empathy, you create a supportive and positive interaction.

When you are in a leadership or team role, transmitting your positive attitude can inspire and motivate those around you. Leading by example, celebrating successes, and maintaining a positive outlook even in the face of setbacks can foster a positive and productive work environment.

Encouraging and uplifting others is also a powerful way to transmit your positive attitude. Offering words of encouragement, recognizing others' achievements, and being a source of inspiration can spread positivity and boost morale.

In your personal life, transmitting your positive attitude can strengthen your relationships and create a supportive network. Whether it is with family, friends, or acquaintances, sharing your positivity can lead to more meaningful and fulfilling connections.

Finally, remember that maintaining a positive attitude is an ongoing effort. It is normal to have off days or face challenges that test your positivity. However, by consistently choosing to focus on the positive, you can develop resilience and continue to transmit your positive attitude to those around you.

In conclusion, transmitting your positive attitude involves effective communication, positive body language, mindful language choices, active listening, leading by example, encouraging others, and maintaining positivity in your personal relationships. By sharing your positivity, you can create a ripple effect that uplifts and inspires those around you, both personally and professionally.

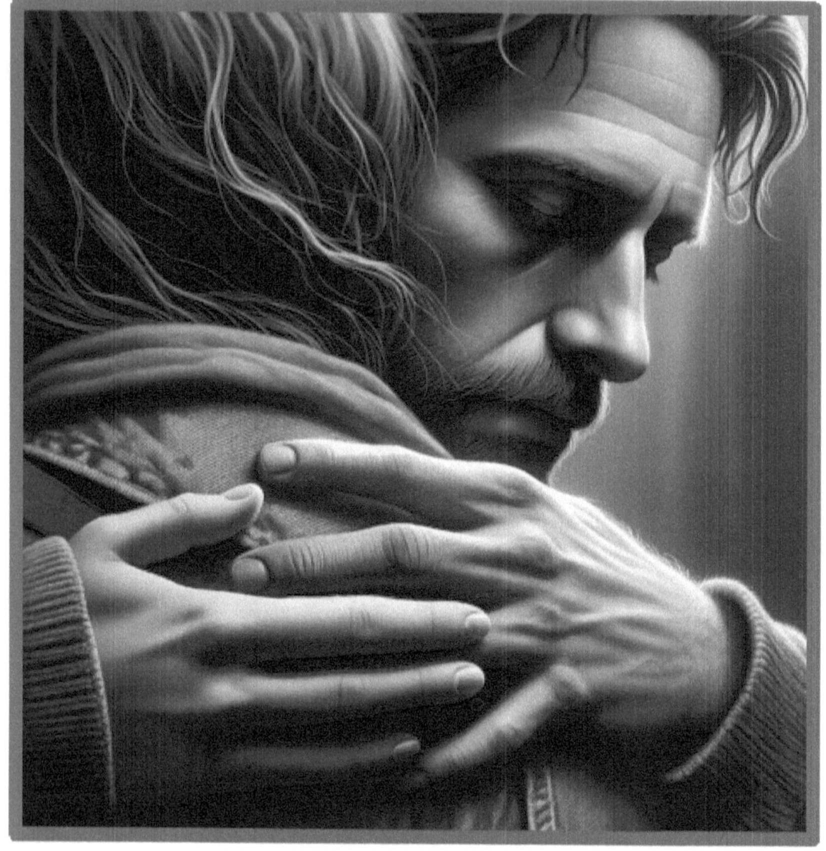

Let People Know You Care

One of the ways you can be more motivated and feel great about yourself on a daily basis is to let people know that you care. Just like the little things in life that you enjoy so much, it is the little things you can do to make others feel great too. You do not have to get credit for these things. You will feel great making someone else feel good. Sometimes you will feel even better doing things for people without them knowing who it is.

When you do things for others, it can be a number of things. You might consider sending token items to friends and family like cards and flowers. Anyone you care about you should always let them know that you care. You do not have to buy items and spend money. If you do not have money to spend, there are other ways to do nice things for people. These things might include something simple like pouring them a cup of coffee, washing their car, or anything else.

Letting people know you care about them is important to them, but it also will make you feel good. You should always let people know that you care, and you appreciate them. There are so many ways you can let people know that you care, and you do not have to spend money either.

In addition to tangible gestures, sometimes a simple conversation can show that you care. Taking the time to ask someone how they are doing, listening to their concerns, and offering words of encouragement can be incredibly meaningful.

Offering your help or assistance in times of need is another way to show you care. Whether it is helping a friend move, assisting a colleague with a project, or lending a hand to a neighbor in need, your willingness to help demonstrates your care and concern for their well-being.

Writing a heartfelt note or letter can also be a powerful way to express your care. In a world where digital communication is prevalent, receiving a handwritten note can feel special and personal.

Celebrating others' achievements and milestones is a way to show you care about their success and happiness. Whether it is a birthday, a promotion, or any other accomplishment, acknowledging these moments shows that you value and appreciate them.

Being present and available is an important aspect of showing care. In times of celebration or in times of sorrow, being there for someone can speak volumes about how much you care.

Practicing empathy and understanding is crucial in letting people know you care. Being able to put yourself in someone else's shoes and offer support and compassion can strengthen your relationships and show that you genuinely care about their experiences.

In conclusion, letting people know you care is about the small, thoughtful actions you take to make others feel valued and appreciated. Whether it is through gestures, words, or simply being present, showing care can have a positive impact on both the giver and the receiver. By making an effort to express your care for others, you not only enhance their lives but also enrich your own.

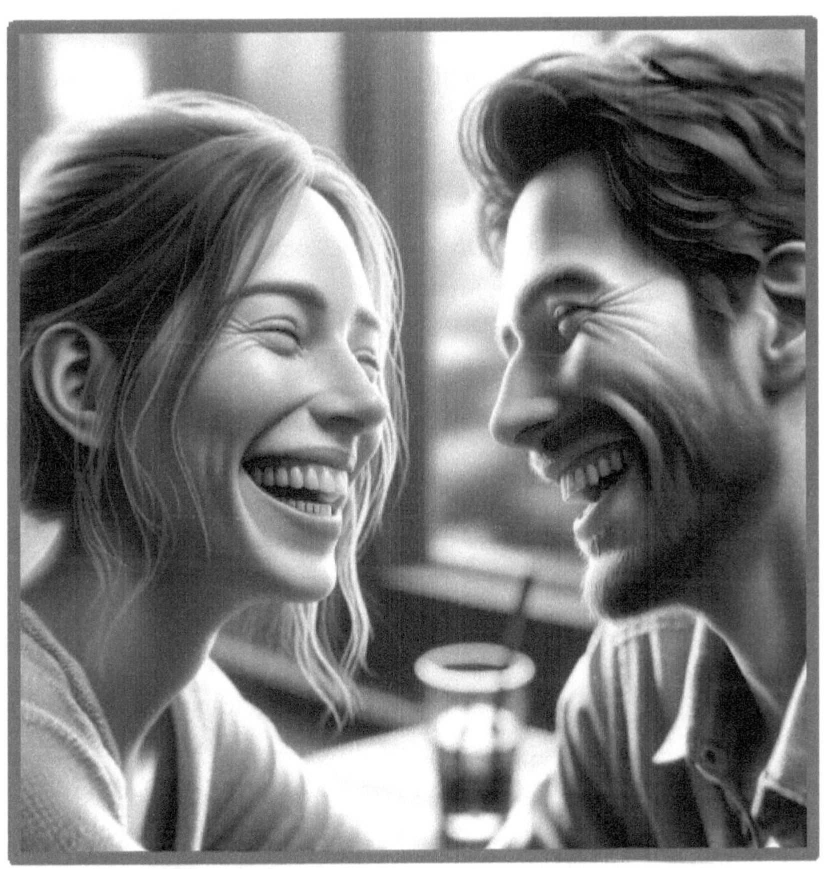

Share Your Sense of Humor

Laughing is healthy for your body and your soul. If you know some funny jokes or you begin to see the funny side of life, you should share this with your friends and people you are around. A sense of humor is good for you, and it is healthy for other people too. The ability to make people laugh is a good thing, and if you are capable of making people laugh, use this skill. This will be good for the people you are making laugh because you are raising their spirits, and it will feel good for you too.

Sharing your sense of humor is good for you and good for the people you are around. You will feel good about yourself and might even be motivated to find new jokes for each day too.

Incorporating humor into your daily interactions can lighten the mood and make even mundane tasks more enjoyable. Whether it is a witty comment during a meeting or a funny observation while running errands, your humor can brighten someone's day.

When sharing your sense of humor, it is important to be mindful of your audience. Different people have different senses of humor, so what is hilarious to one person might not be as funny to another. Being sensitive to others' preferences and boundaries is key to sharing humor effectively.

Using humor can also be a great way to diffuse tense situations. A well-timed joke or humorous remark can break the ice and ease tension, making it easier to navigate challenging conversations or stressful moments.

Sharing humorous stories or experiences is another way to connect with others. Laughing together over a funny incident can create a sense of camaraderie and strengthen your relationships.

In the workplace, a sense of humor can be a valuable asset. It can help build rapport with colleagues, foster a positive work environment, and make you more approachable.

Incorporating humor into presentations or speeches can make them more engaging and memorable. A good laugh can capture your audience's attention and make your message more relatable.

It is also important to use humor appropriately. Avoid jokes that are offensive, insensitive, or inappropriate for the situation. The goal is to bring joy and laughter, not discomfort or offense.

In conclusion, sharing your sense of humor is a wonderful way to spread joy and positivity. It is good for your well-being and can have a positive impact on those around you. By using humor thoughtfully and considerately, you can create moments of laughter and light-heartedness that enrich your life and the lives of others.

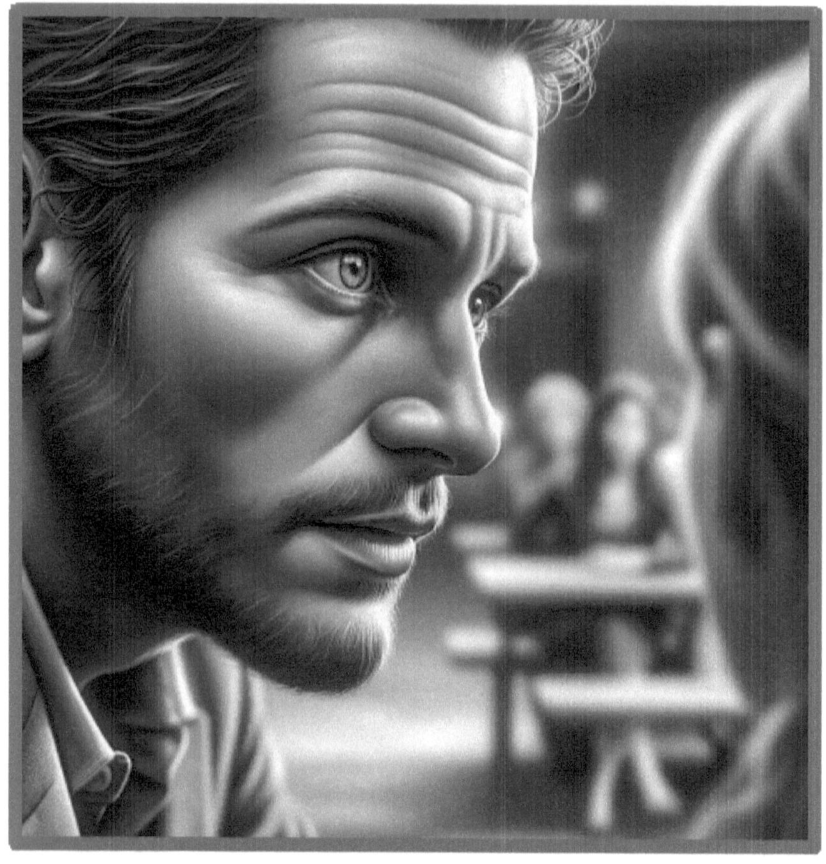

Be a Good Listener

Helping others create motivation and a positive attitude also means you need to be a good listener. When you listen to people, they realize you actually care about what they have to say. It shows you have a sensitive side too. When you listen to others, they realize that they have something positive to focus on.

Listening to people gives you the opportunity to show people the positive in the negative they are focusing on. This will help you help them. Listening means understanding how the person is feeling about what they are saying. You might want to repeat back to the person some of the things they are saying. This will reinforce to the person you are listening to that you are listening to them. When you are a good listener, it will make you feel great because you will see the positive effect it has on the other person. You will also create a better friend too.

Being a good listener involves more than just hearing the words someone is saying. It requires active engagement and genuine interest in the other person's thoughts and feelings. By giving your full attention and avoiding distractions, you show that you value the conversation and the person with whom you are communicating.

Asking open-ended questions is another way to be a good listener. This encourages the speaker to share more about their experiences and feelings, and it shows that you are interested in understanding their perspective.

Empathy is a crucial component of being a good listener. By putting yourself in the other person's shoes and acknowledging their emotions, you can provide comfort and support. Empathy helps build trust and strengthens your connection with the person you are listening to.

It is also important to avoid interrupting or offering unsolicited advice. Sometimes, people just need to express themselves without looking for solutions. By refraining from jumping in with your own opinions or solutions, you allow the speaker to fully express themselves and feel heard.

Practicing patience is essential when listening. Some people may take longer to articulate their thoughts or may need time to process their emotions. By being patient, you create a safe space for them to express themselves at their own pace.

Being a good listener also means being non-judgmental. Avoiding judgment and criticism encourages open and honest communication. When people feel safe to share without fear of judgment, they are more likely to open up and share their true thoughts and feelings.

In conclusion, being a good listener is a valuable skill that can enhance your relationships and help others feel valued and understood.

By giving your full attention, asking open-ended questions, showing empathy, avoiding interruptions, practicing patience, and being non-judgmental, you can become a better listener and a more supportive friend or confidant. This not only benefits the people you listen to but also enriches your own life by fostering deeper connections and a greater sense of empathy.

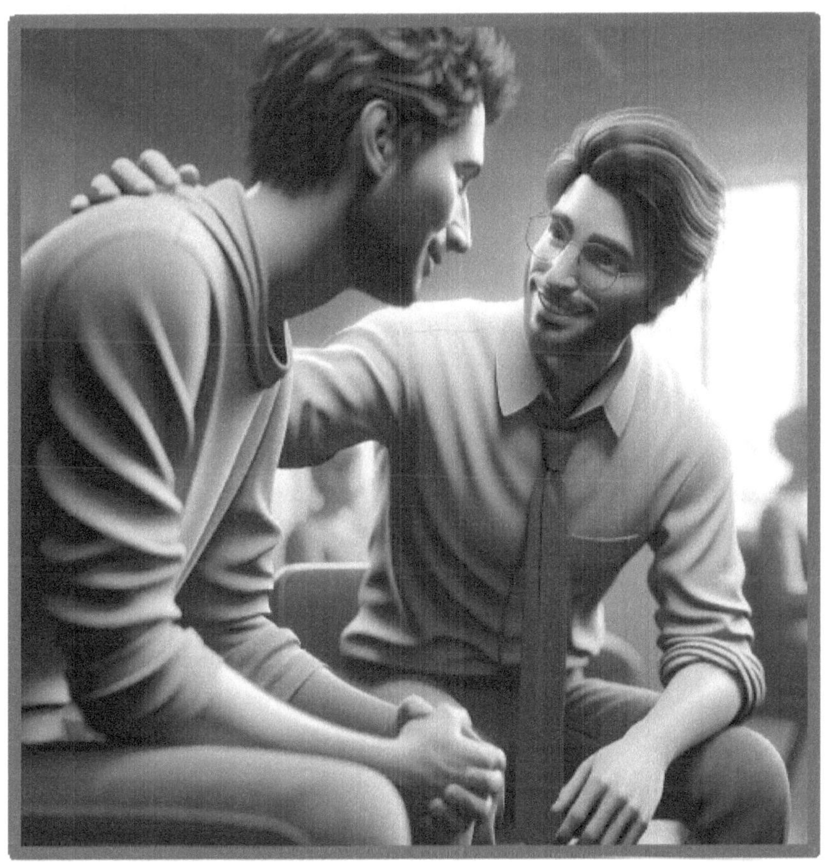

Give Your Positive Attitude

There are many ways you can give a positive attitude to other people. Many of the other people include laughing, paying compliments, and setting an example.

Laughing is contagious. People are often drawn to laughter, and they want to take part in the fun. Laughing is also healthy too. You might find people who laugh often really are happy and healthy individuals. You should share your laugh and your attitude will be very infectious to the people around you. You will feel good about yourself also.

Communicating your positive attitude can be done through a positive attitude and the best way to convey that is through paying compliments to people. When you see the positive side in others always feel free to share this with them. Notice someone's nice hat or shoes. People love compliments and it gives them a boost and will make you feel better about yourself also.

Another way to give your positive attitude to other people is by setting an example. When you do good things and people around you see it, they will jump in and help too. This includes stopping along the side of the road and helping someone change a tire on the car. You might see someone at work in a break room cleaning up a mess from a luncheon. When you give your positive attitude, and you are not afraid to give it to other people who will join in.

There are many things that you can do to help others. When you help others with your positive attitude and behaviors it will feel great. You will be motivated to help others. By following these many different techniques, you will find you are much more motivated each day to complete certain tasks and you will be creating an environment that is positive with all of the people around you.

In addition to laughter, compliments, and setting an example, you can also give your positive attitude by being supportive. Offering encouragement and support to friends, family, and colleagues can boost their confidence and help them overcome challenges.

Showing gratitude is another way to spread positivity. Expressing appreciation for the people and things in your life can inspire others to do the same and foster a more positive environment.

Being kind and considerate in your interactions can also convey a positive attitude. Simple acts of kindness, like holding the door open for someone or offering a helping hand, can make a big difference in someone's day.

Listening attentively and showing empathy is another way to give your positive attitude. By genuinely caring about others' feelings and perspectives, you create a positive and supportive atmosphere.

Maintaining a positive outlook even in difficult situations can also influence those around you. When you face challenges with optimism and resilience, it can encourage others to adopt a similar attitude.

In conclusion, giving your positive attitude involves a combination of laughter, compliments, setting an example, being supportive, showing gratitude, being kind, listening attentively, and maintaining a positive outlook. By embodying these qualities and sharing them with others, you can spread positivity and make a positive impact on the people around you. This not only enhances your own well-being but also contributes to a more positive and supportive community.

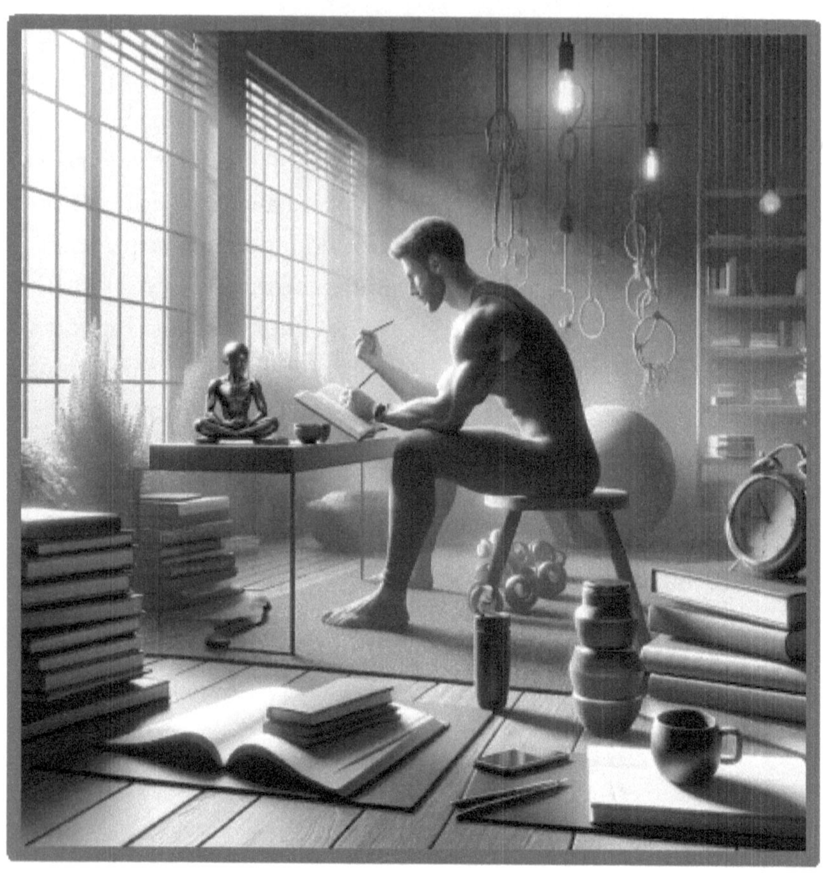

Chapter 10 – Building Motivational Habits

There are many ways you can build motivational habits on a daily basis. Habits can be hard to create but once you begin working hard to meet them, they will begin to come naturally to you. There are many things you can do to create habits that are motivating and positive.

One of the first steps in building motivational habits is setting clear and achievable goals. Having specific goals gives you a direction and a sense of purpose. Break down your goals into smaller, manageable tasks, and celebrate each accomplishment along the way. This will help you maintain motivation and momentum.

Creating a routine is another important aspect of building motivational habits. Establishing a daily or weekly schedule that includes time for work, rest, and activities you enjoy can help you stay organized and focused. Consistency is key, so try to stick to your routine as much as possible.

Surrounding yourself with positivity is also crucial. This can mean surrounding yourself with positive people who encourage and support you, as well as creating a positive environment. Decorate your workspace with inspirational quotes or images, listen to uplifting music, or read motivational books to keep your spirits high.

Practicing gratitude is a powerful motivational habit. Take time each day to reflect on the things you are thankful for. This can help shift your focus from what you lack to what you have, fostering a positive mindset that can drive motivation.

Visualization is another effective tool for building motivational habits. Spend a few minutes each day visualizing yourself achieving your goals. Imagine the sense of accomplishment and the positive emotions associated with success. This mental rehearsal can boost your confidence and motivation.

Self-discipline is essential for maintaining motivational habits. There will be days when you do not want to stick to your routine or working towards your goals. It is during these times that self-discipline becomes crucial. Remind yourself of the bigger picture and the reasons behind your goals to keep yourself on track.

Rewarding yourself for your achievements is also important. When you reach a milestone or complete a task, treat yourself to something you enjoy. This positive reinforcement can increase your motivation to continue working towards your goals.

Staying adaptable and open to change is also important. Sometimes, despite your best efforts, things may not go as planned. Being able to adjust your goals, routines, or strategies can help you stay motivated in the face of challenges.

Lastly, remember that building motivational habits is a journey, not a destination. It is about making continuous improvements and learning from your experiences. Be patient with yourself and recognize that every step forward is progress.

In conclusion, building motivational habits involves setting goals, creating a routine, surrounding yourself with positivity, practicing gratitude, visualizing success, exercising self-discipline, rewarding achievements, staying adaptable, and embracing the journey. By incorporating these habits into your daily life, you can cultivate a motivational mindset that propels you towards your goals and aspirations.

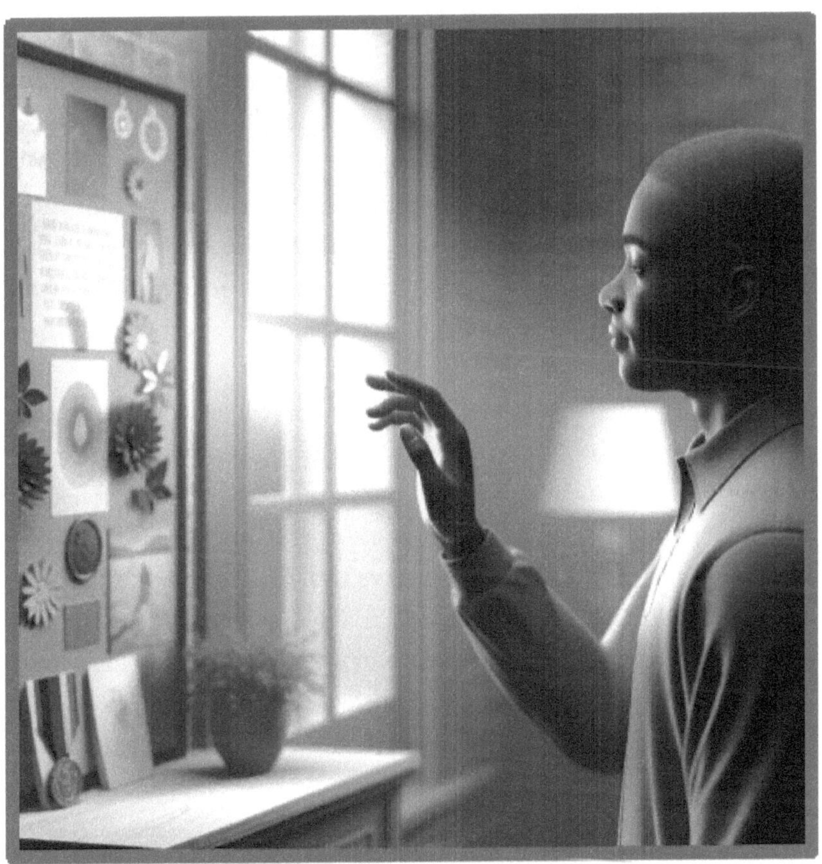

Visual Motivators

Visual motivators are extremely important because your surroundings can create the attitude you have every day. If you are in a negative atmosphere, you will not feel motivated to do much at all. One thing you can do is use visual motivators to create a positive atmosphere and help you on a daily basis.

Visual motivators are things that include positive quotes for you to read and focus on. They might include a change you hope to make in your life. There are many posters you can choose from to post on your walls or cubicle in your home. This way, you can read them and focus on the positive on these positive statements.

If you do not want to paste these things on your walls, you might consider a motivational calendar. Every day the calendar will give you a new quote to focus on for the day. Some people like to use cartoons and jokes to maintain a good attitude.

There are many things you might consider to be a visual motivator. These things include anything that makes you feel really good and positive. Remember that visual motivators are to be used to motivate you on a daily basis because they will be somewhere you will see them every day.

In addition to quotes and calendars, you can also use images or photographs as visual motivators. Pictures of your goals, such as a dream vacation destination or a fitness aspiration, can serve as a constant reminder of what you are working towards.

Vision boards are another effective tool for visual motivation. By creating a collage of images, quotes, and symbols that represent your aspirations, you can keep your goals visually present in your daily life.

You can also personalize your workspace or living area with objects that inspire you. This could be anything from a souvenir from a memorable trip, a trophy or medal from an achievement, or even a plant that adds life and energy to your space.

Setting up your environment to reflect your goals and aspirations can also serve as a visual motivator. For example, if you are aiming to read more books, having a well-organized bookshelf in a prominent place can encourage you to reach for a book more often.

Digital visual motivators can also be impactful. Changing your computer or phone wallpaper to an image or quote that inspires you can be a simple yet effective way to keep motivation at your fingertips.

In conclusion, visual motivators are a powerful tool to help create and maintain a positive and motivated mindset. By surrounding yourself with images, quotes, and objects that inspire you, you can keep your goals and aspirations front and center, providing a constant source of motivation to pursue your dreams.

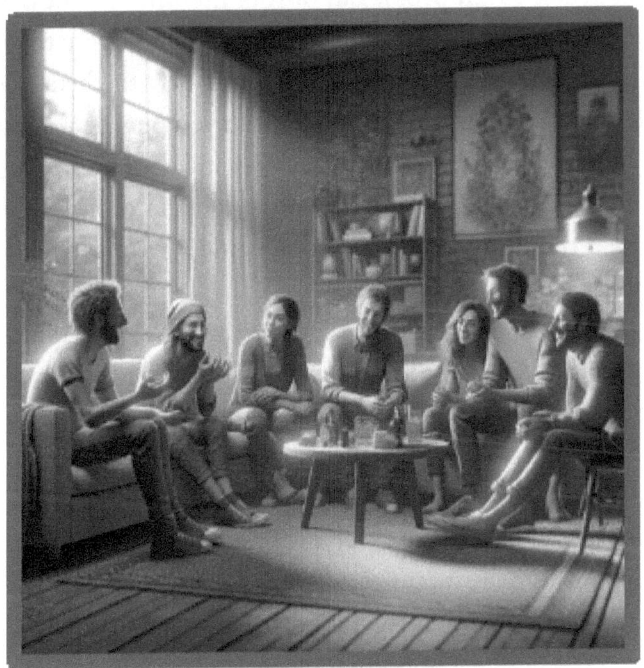

Maintain Positive Friends

Friends are people you have a good relationship with and people who care about you. Those people will always build you up and make you feel good.

If you have a friend that shoots you down or makes you feel negative all of the time, then you should not maintain them as a friend. Always spend time with the people who make you feel good about life and good about yourself. The more time you spend around people who make you feel good, the better you will feel.

It is true that you become the people you spend time together with. If the people you spend time together with only put you down and do not support the things that are important to you, it will be too hard for you to become the motivated person you want to be. You need a support group that is positive.

If you decide to cut people out of your life who are not positive or help you, it might be difficult for you. You might choose to gradually stop talking to them or you might try and talk to them about the negativity. If their friendship means a lot to you, maybe you can point out the negativity and see how they respond. Some people do not realize they are being so negative until someone points it out. This could save a friendship and maybe you could have a partner to begin the quest for motivation together.

In addition to cutting out negative influences, it is important to actively seek out and nurture friendships with positive people. Surrounding yourself with individuals who are optimistic, supportive, and encouraging can significantly impact your own outlook and motivation.

Positive friends can also serve as role models and sources of inspiration. Seeing the successes and positive attitudes of those around you can motivate you to pursue your own goals and maintain a positive mindset.

It is also beneficial to engage in activities that promote positivity with your friends. Whether it is participating in a hobby you all enjoy, volunteering together, or simply having regular get-togethers to share good news and celebrate achievements, these shared experiences can strengthen your bond and reinforce a positive outlook.

Open communication is key to maintaining positive friendships. Being able to express your thoughts, feelings, and aspirations openly and receiving supportive feedback can create a strong foundation for a lasting and positive relationship.

Lastly, remember that maintaining positive friendships is a two-way street. Just as you seek out friends who uplift you, strive to be a positive influence in the lives of your friends. By offering support, encouragement, and positivity, you can contribute to a mutually beneficial and uplifting friendship.

In conclusion, maintaining positive friends is crucial for your overall well-being and motivation. By surrounding yourself with supportive and optimistic individuals, actively nurturing those relationships, and being a positive influence yourself, you can create a network of friends that enhances your life and helps you achieve your goals.

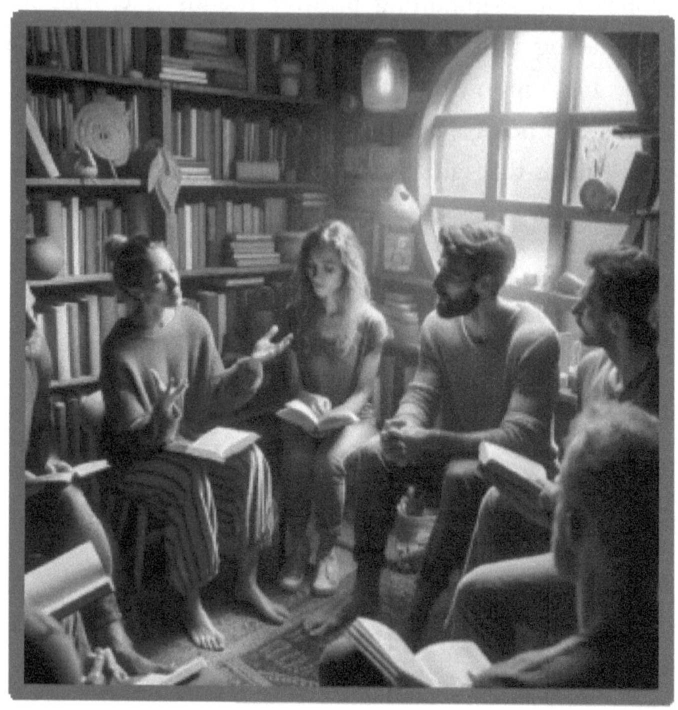

Read and Listen

Reading and listening are two habits you must build for your motivational daily routine. Reading is the best thing you can do to strengthen your mind and build confidence. In order to become the person, you strive to be, you must read about how to be this person. You need to associate with people you admire and want to be like to form these habits. It is quite common that you become a mixture of the people you associate with because you pick up the habits.

Reading provides a wealth of knowledge and insights that can inspire and motivate you. It can expose you to new ideas, different perspectives, and success stories that can fuel your motivation. Whether it is self-help books, biographies of successful individuals, or literature that challenges your thinking, reading can be a powerful tool for personal growth.

Listening is equally important in your motivational journey. Listening to podcasts, audiobooks, or engaging in conversations with mentors and like-minded individuals can provide valuable lessons and encouragement. Active listening allows you to absorb information, learn from others' experiences, and apply that knowledge to your own life.

Incorporating reading and listening into your daily routine does not have to be overwhelming. Setting aside a specific time each day for these activities can help you develop a consistent habit. Even just 15-30 minutes of focused reading or listening can make a significant difference over time.

When choosing what to read or listen to, select materials that align with your goals and interests. This will keep you engaged and ensure that the information is relevant to your personal development journey.

Taking notes or highlighting key points while reading or listening can help you retain and reflect on the information. This practice can also aid in identifying actionable steps you can take to implement the ideas into your life.

Discussing what you have read or listened to with others can further enhance your understanding and provide different viewpoints. Engaging in conversations about the material can deepen your insights and motivate you to take action.

It is also important to be open-minded and willing to explore a variety of genres and topics. Diversifying your reading and listening materials can broaden your knowledge base and introduce you to new concepts that can enrich your life.

In conclusion, reading and listening are essential habits for building motivation and achieving personal growth. By dedicating time to these activities, selecting materials that align with your goals, and actively engaging with the content, you can strengthen your mind, build confidence, and become the person you strive to be. Surrounding yourself with positive influences and continually seeking knowledge will propel you forward on your motivational journey.

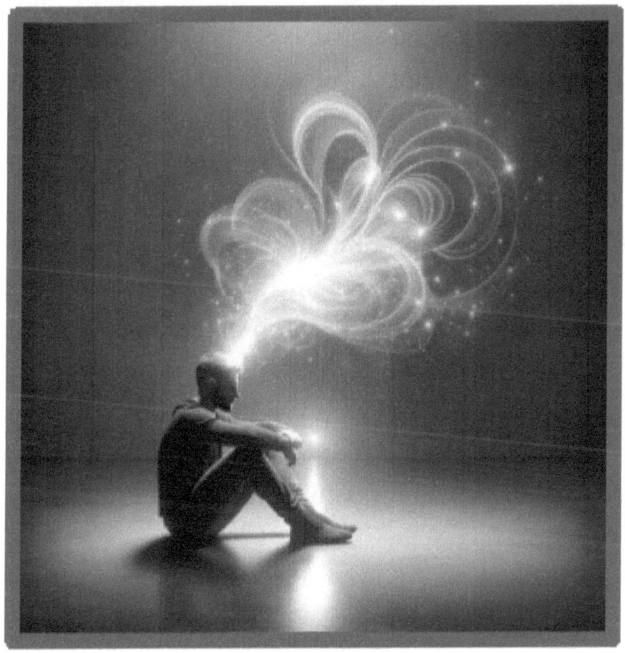

Self-Talk

Positive self-talk is an especially important daily habit you need to build. There will be circumstances you need to walk yourself through, and positive talk will help you make it through these times. Self-talk can help you in many ways. It can help you feel good about yourself, how you look, and how you are going to perform at a certain event.

If you have a meeting, you are extremely nervous about it because you have to give a presentation, positive self-talk can help with encouraging yourself to do a good job. It is not crazy to talk yourself through situations.

As you would feed off positive reinforcement through others, you can stroke these needs also. When you wake up in the morning and you need to give yourself a little encouragement, there is nothing wrong with talking to yourself about making it through the events of the day. Create the positive circumstances in your head and make them happen.

When you talk to yourself positively, you will begin to believe in the positive and act positively.

Practicing positive self-talk involves replacing negative thoughts with positive affirmations. Instead of thinking, "I can't do this," tell yourself, "I can handle this challenge." This shift in mindset can have a profound impact on your confidence and motivation.

It is also important to be kind and compassionate to yourself. Treat yourself with the same understanding and support you would offer a friend. Acknowledge your efforts and progress, even if things are not perfect.

Positive self-talk can also help you manage stress and anxiety. By focusing on positive outcomes and reassuring yourself that you can cope with difficult situations, you can reduce feelings of stress and increase your resilience.

Visualization can be a powerful tool in conjunction with positive self-talk. Visualizing yourself succeeding in a task or achieving a goal can reinforce your belief in your abilities and increase your motivation to take action.

Regularly practicing positive self-talk can lead to a more optimistic outlook on life. Over time, it can become a natural part of your thought process, helping you to maintain a positive attitude even in challenging situations.

It is important to be aware of your inner dialogue and actively work on making it more positive. This might involve monitoring your thoughts and consciously replacing negative self-talk with positive affirmations.

Positive self-talk is not about denying reality or ignoring problems. It is about approaching life with a positive mindset and believing in your ability to overcome obstacles.

In conclusion, positive self-talk is a vital habit for personal growth and motivation. By regularly engaging in positive self-talk, you can boost your confidence, reduce stress, and cultivate a more positive outlook on life. Remember to be kind to yourself, focus on positive outcomes, and believe in your ability to succeed.

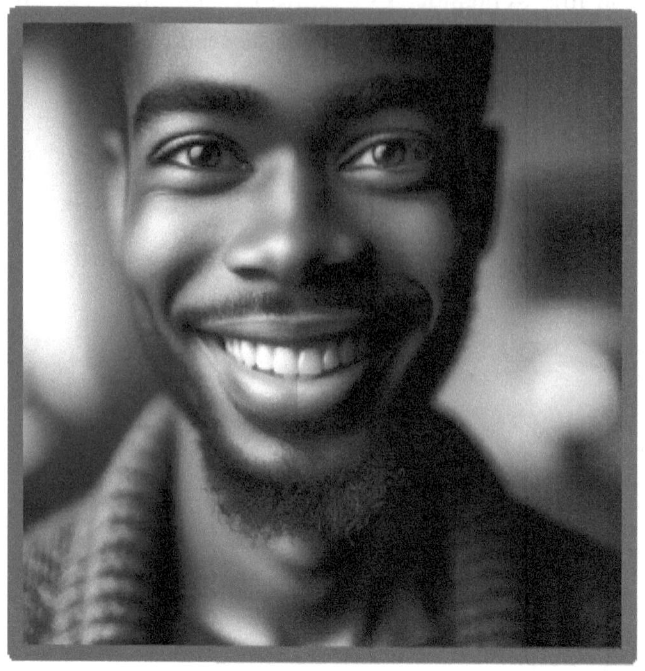

Maintain a Positive Attitude

You must remain positive. Life is tough and you need to get used to it. As soon as you stop thinking life is so difficult, you will find it becomes so much easier. Do not focus on how difficult life is. Dealing with the difficulties of life.

A positive attitude is vital to make it through your days and be motivated. When you are positive about certain events and circumstances that you often deem too tough, you will make it through the obstacles much easier.

The most important thing you need to remember about your attitude is that once you realize you cannot choose and control the circumstances, you do have total control over the attitude toward circumstances you face. You can maintain a positive attitude. A positive attitude will help you feel so much better about certain circumstances as you come across them and they will not feel so difficult.

Maintaining a positive attitude also involves focusing on solutions rather than problems. Instead of dwelling on what is going wrong, shift your attention to finding ways to make things right. This proactive approach can help you feel more empowered and less overwhelmed.

Gratitude is another key component of a positive attitude. Regularly acknowledging the good things in your life, no matter how small, can shift your perspective and help you appreciate the positive aspects of any situation.

Surrounding yourself with positive influences can also reinforce your positive attitude. Seek out friends, family members, and colleagues who uplift you and encourage your positive outlook.

It is also important to practice self-care to maintain a positive attitude. Taking care of your physical and mental health through regular exercise, healthy eating, and adequate rest can boost your mood and resilience.

Positive affirmations can be a powerful tool to reinforce a positive attitude. Repeating positive statements to yourself, such as "I am capable of overcoming challenges" or "I am worthy of happiness," can help you internalize these beliefs and approach life with a more positive mindset.

Remember that maintaining a positive attitude does not mean ignoring negative emotions or pretending everything is okay when it is not. It is about acknowledging challenges while choosing to focus on the positive and believing in your ability to overcome obstacles.

In conclusion, maintaining a positive attitude is essential for navigating life's challenges and staying motivated. By focusing on solutions, practicing gratitude, surrounding yourself with positivity, taking care of yourself, and using affirmations, you can cultivate a positive outlook that will help you face difficulties with confidence and resilience.

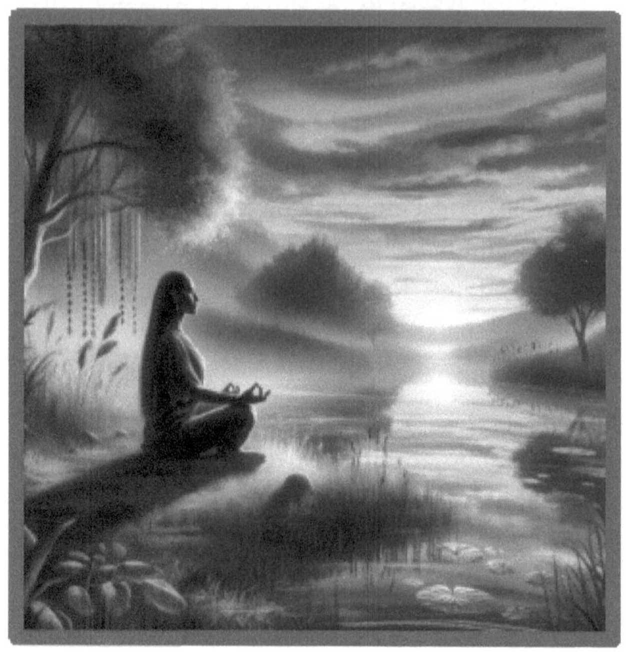

Breaks

One of the things to remember is that you need to slow down every now and then and take a break. Give yourself the time to reload the energy and recharge your batteries. Taking a break means giving yourself a moment to relax. This does not mean getting caught up in a realm of procrastination. If you have a bad habit of getting drawn into a television, then do not take a break in front of the TV. Be sure the break you take is for a short while but does not lead to a problem.

If you have a big family and the house is often chaotic, the 'me' time is especially important. Chances are good you have to wait until all of the children are asleep or early in the morning before they wake up. If you have to schedule this time for yourself, you should. You will be surprised how amazing just a little bit of time to yourself each day will help you feel more motivated to face situations.

Taking breaks is not just about resting; it is also about giving your mind a chance to refresh and gain new perspectives. When you step away from your tasks, you allow yourself to return with renewed focus and creativity.

It is important to find activities that truly relax you during your breaks. This could be anything from reading a book, going for a walk, practicing meditation, or simply sitting quietly and enjoying a cup of tea. The key is to engage in activities that help you unwind and detach from the demands of your day.

Breaks can also be an opportunity to engage in physical activity. Exercise is not only beneficial for your physical health but also for your mental well-being. A short walk or a quick workout session can boost your energy levels and improve your mood.

Incorporating regular breaks into your daily routine can help prevent burnout. When you work without sufficient rest, your productivity and motivation can suffer. By taking breaks, you ensure that you stay sharp and engaged in your tasks.

It is also important to set boundaries during your breaks. If possible, disconnect from work-related emails or messages. This helps you fully enjoy your break and return to your tasks with a clearer mind.

Remember, taking breaks is not a sign of weakness or laziness. It is a crucial aspect of maintaining your overall well-being and enhancing your productivity. By giving yourself permission to take breaks, you are investing in your long-term success and happiness.

In conclusion, breaks are an essential part of maintaining motivation and overall well-being. By taking the time to relax and recharge, you can improve your focus, creativity, and productivity. Whether it is a few minutes of quiet time, a short walk, or engaging in a relaxing activity, make sure to incorporate regular breaks into your routine to stay motivated and energized.

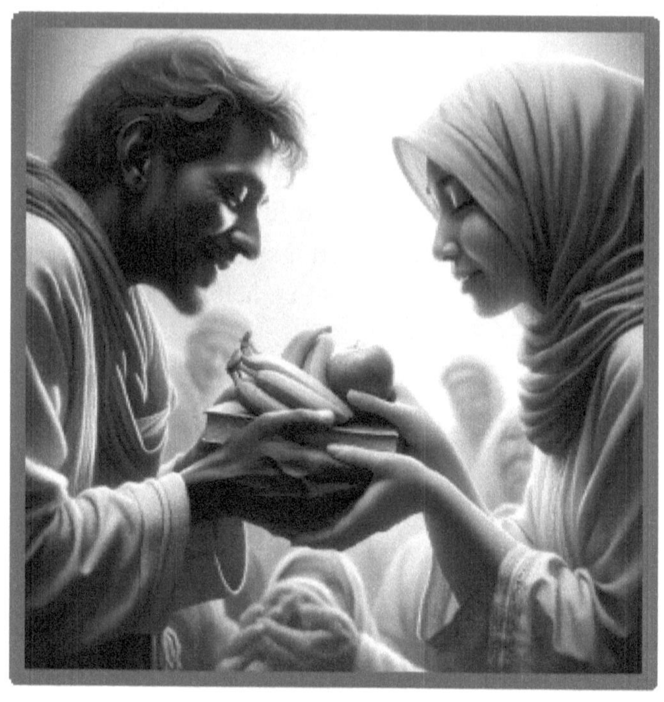

Share with Others

Once you have become motivated, you can begin to share your motivation with others. When you share motivation, it will be contagious, and so will your passion. As you share your passions, you will also find that you are now driven to new heights of goals and accomplishments. Be sure to share your motivation on a daily basis. This part of your daily regimen of motivation may not be something you do right away because you need to work on you first.

Sharing your motivation can take many forms. It could be as simple as sharing an inspiring quote with a friend, offering words of encouragement to a colleague, or sharing your personal success stories with others. When you share your motivation, you not only inspire others but also reinforce your own commitment to your goals.

You can also share your motivation by being a role model. Leading by example is a powerful way to motivate others. When people see you actively pursuing your goals, staying positive, and overcoming challenges, they are more likely to be inspired to do the same.

Another way to share your motivation is through mentorship or coaching. If you have the opportunity to mentor someone, use it as a chance to share your knowledge, experiences, and motivational strategies. Helping someone else achieve their goals can be incredibly rewarding and can further fuel your own motivation.

Sharing your motivation can also involve creating or joining a support group or community. Being part of a group of like-minded individuals who are all working towards their goals can provide a sense of camaraderie and accountability. It is a great way to stay motivated and help others stay motivated as well.

It is important to remember that everyone's motivation is unique. What motivates you might not necessarily motivate someone else. When sharing your motivation, be respectful of others' perspectives and be open to learning from their experiences as well.

Sharing your motivation is not just about inspiring others; it is also about creating a positive environment around you. When you surround yourself with motivated individuals, it creates a feedback loop of positivity and encouragement that benefits everyone involved.

Finally, remember that sharing your motivation is an ongoing process. It is not something about which you do once and then forget. Continuously sharing your motivation, celebrating successes, and encouraging others through their challenges can help build a supportive and motivated community.

In conclusion, sharing your motivation with others is a crucial aspect of maintaining your own motivation and inspiring those around you. By sharing your passion, being a role model, offering mentorship, and creating a supportive community, you can spread motivation and positivity. This not only helps others achieve their goals but also enhances your own journey towards success.

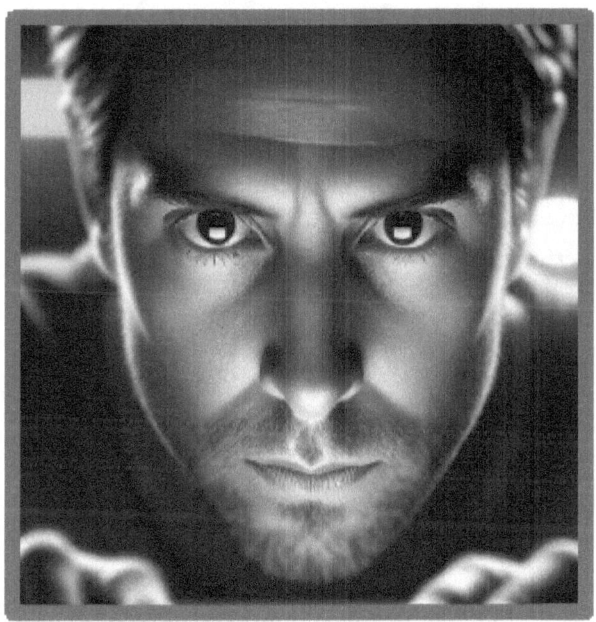

Chapter 11 – Maximizing Motivation

As you become motivated there are certain techniques you can also use on a daily basis for yourself to maximize the motivation and make you feel great. Many of the things you need to consider include consequences, pleasure, instructions, incentives and more.

Consequences are something to think about when it comes to maximizing your motivation. You can think about the consequences and even point them out if you are trying to motivate others for a good performance. It is important to remember not to use consequences as threats. Threats will cause people to turn against you. There is a big difference between awareness and threats. For self-motivation, the knowing the consequences can help someone become organized.

Incentives and rewards are especially important. You might never treat yourself to something good and it is time you did. Self-reward is one of the best ways to get motivated. Go buy that new watch you have had your eyes on for some time. Be sure it is after you reach that goal you are working toward.

Instructions are also an important way to get the best out of your motivational techniques. You might find that you can never rely on anyone because they always let you down. Maybe they did not understand. Instructions should be detailed and clear. Do not make someone feel like a child but you can provide instructions to help people make it through an expectation.

Most people work better when they know what you expect from them. You might need to write down instructions for yourself also. Never take on a project if you are not sure about how to complete it. If there are questions about the steps involved always be sure to ask questions. Clarity on specific projects will help you become more motivated to make it to the completion date.

Setting goals for your process of action. These goals should be short term and long term. Be clear on which goals are realistically reachable in a short-term time and which goals may take years to achieve. Goals can help you guide the process of action and help you create philosophies in your life. Goals are motivating and must always be set. When you stop goal setting you will no longer be motivated to achieve anything.

Trust and respect are also two other things you must consider. People need to be trusted and respected and when they know they have these two things from you they will respond to you in a better way. If you are trying to motivate others, you need to give people trust and respect because they will want to do things for you.

Constructive criticism is also especially important for maximizing motivation. If you are trying to motivate others, you should always be constructive and not damaging.

Beating someone down will not help them become motivated but it will cause the situation to possibly turn into a bad one.

When you provide constructive criticism, you can still see the positive outcome of the circumstance and you can also help people find positive ways to remedy situations. This includes you too. Never beat yourself up. On a daily basis you need to bring positive reinforcement and also constructive criticism. Do not be hard on yourself. Remember, life is tougher for someone else out there.

Make life fun. When you work on projects in your personal life and at work you need to find the fun in all of the processes. Making things fun can help motivate others who are having a hard time making it through. If your work does not feel like work, you will enjoy it so much more. If your employees are lacking motivation, then make it a fun and positive environment. This will lead to excellent results with the staff rather than problems with hostility.

Communication is another way to remain motivated and to motivate others. You need to be sure all communication lines are open and there is never a disconnect. If there are any potential problems that could arise you need to be aware of everything that could happen. The more aware you are of issues that could arise the less severe it seems when they happen. Awareness can also help you prevent things from occurring too.

Stimulation is important to. Be sure each day you practice something that is stimulating for you. Stimulation is good for the brain and to remain motivated. If you do the same thing every single day you will become bored, find it hard to reach goals, and lack motivation. Be sure you create a stimulating environment for yourself or just mix things up a bit. All you have to do is change things up a bit. It can help you be enthusiastic and also have the opportunity to see the big picture in life too.

Improvements are important. One thing you need to add to your motivational guide is to demand improvements. As you practice your motivational techniques you can find ways to improve your attitude and the way you do things. You can find specific areas where you can improve and make them better. As you see these areas you can create a focal point and set goals too. This will help keep you motivated to work toward these goals.

Demanding improvement is an excellent way to avoid stagnation with you and in others. When people improve or you improve do not be afraid to raise the bar. This helps people excel even further beyond what you or others might have thought you could have done.

You should also create opportunities for you or others to maximize motivation. If you do not see an opportunity to advance, then you need to find one. This means creating an opportunity. This means you can become motivated when you see the

opportunities in things that you can achieve. This also means you need to provide or create opportunities for employees too. When you are aware of how your hard work can actually create a payoff, you will be more motivated. Motivation works great when there is an opportunity sitting in front of someone.

Another thing to think about is being creative. When you work on your motivational techniques every day be sure you are creative. Never be afraid to use your creative side. If you are used to getting shot down when you are creative ignore these things. It is healthy to be creative. Encourage As you become motivated, there are certain techniques you can also use on a daily basis for yourself to maximize the motivation and make you feel great. Many of the things you need to consider include consequences, pleasure, instructions, incentives, and more.

Consequences are something to think about when it comes to maximizing your motivation. You can think about the consequences and even point them out if you are trying to motivate others for a good performance. It is important to remember not to use consequences as threats. Threats will cause people to turn against you. There is a big difference between awareness and threats. For self-motivation, knowing the consequences can help someone become organized.

Incentives and rewards are especially important. You might never treat yourself to something good and it is time you did. Self-reward is one of the best ways to get motivated. Go buy that new watch you have had your eyes on for some time. Be sure it is after you reach that goal you are working toward.

Instructions are also an important way to get the best out of your motivational techniques. You might find that you can never rely on anyone because they always let you down. Maybe they did not understand. Instructions should be detailed and clear. Do not make someone feel like a child but you can provide instructions to help people make it through an expectation.

Most people work better when they know what you expect from them. You might need to write down instructions for yourself also. Never take on a project if you are not sure about how to complete it. If there are questions about the steps involved always be sure to ask questions. Clarity on specific projects will help you become more motivated to make it to the completion date.

Setting goals for your process of action. These goals should be short-term and long-term. Be clear on which goals are realistically reachable in a short-term time and which goals may take years to achieve. Goals can help you guide the process of action and help you create philosophies in your life. Goals are motivating and must always be set. When you stop goal setting you will no longer be motivated to achieve anything.

Trust and respect are also two other things you must consider. People need to be trusted and respected and when they know they have these two things from you they will respond to you in a better way. If you are trying to motivate others, you need to give people trust and respect because they will want to do things for you.

Constructive criticism is also especially important for maximizing motivation. If you are trying to motivate others, you should always be constructive and not damaging.

Beating someone down will not help them become motivated but it will cause the situation to possibly turn into a bad one.

When you provide constructive criticism, you can still see the positive outcome of the circumstance and you can also help people find positive ways to remedy situations. This includes you too. Never beat yourself up. On a daily basis, you need to bring positive reinforcement and also constructive criticism. Do not be hard on yourself. Remember, life is tougher for someone else out there.

Make life fun. When you work on projects in your personal life and at work you need to find the fun in all of the processes. Making things fun can help motivate others who are having a hard time making it through. If your work does not feel like work, you will enjoy it so much more. If your employees are lacking motivation, then make it a fun and positive environment. This will lead to excellent results with the staff rather than problems with hostility.

Communication is another way to remain motivated and to motivate others. You need to be sure all communication lines are open and there is never a disconnect. If there are any potential problems that could arise you need to be aware of everything that could happen. The more aware you are of issues that could arise the less severe it seems when they happen. Awareness can also help you prevent things from occurring too.

Stimulation is important too. Be sure each day you practice something that is stimulating for you. Stimulation is good for the brain and to remain motivated. If you do the same thing every single day you will become bored, find it hard to reach goals, and lack motivation. Be sure you create a stimulating environment for yourself or just mix things up a bit. All you have to do is change things up a bit. It can help you be enthusiastic and also have the opportunity to see the big picture in life too.

Improvements are important. One thing you need to add to your motivational guide is to demand improvements. As you practice your motivational techniques you can find ways to improve your attitude and the way you do things. You can find specific areas where you can improve and make them better. As you see these areas you can create a focal point and set goals too. This will help keep you motivated to work toward these goals.

Demanding improvement is an excellent way to avoid stagnation with you and in others. When people improve or you improve do not be afraid to raise the bar. This helps people excel even further beyond what you or others might have thought you could have done.

You should also create opportunities for you or others to maximize motivation. If you do not see an opportunity to advance, then you need to find one. This means creating an opportunity. This means you can become motivated when you see the opportunities in things that you can achieve. This also means you need to provide or create opportunities for employees too. When you are aware of how your hard work can actually create a payoff, you will be more motivated. Motivation works great when there is an opportunity sitting in front of someone.

Another thing to think about is being creative. When you work on your motivational techniques every day be sure you are creative. Never be afraid to use your creative side. If you are used to getting shot down when you are creative ignore these things. It is healthy to be creative. Encourage creativity in others too. Some people have a lot they can teach you when you show them you are interested in seeing their creative side, getting creativity in others too. Some people have a lot they can teach you when you show them you are interested in seeing their creative side.

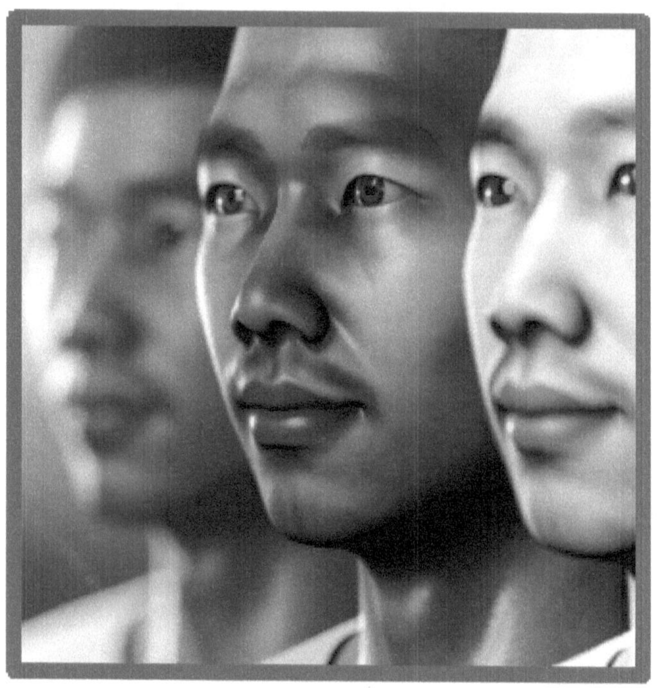

Chapter 12- Conclusion

If you find that you are having a hard time being motivated to make it through the day or certain projects on a regular basis, there are certain things you can do. Motivation includes a combination of behaviors so you can feel the spark to accomplish certain goals and other things.

If you are motivated, you have the oomph you need to make it through anything. There are many things you need to do if you are lacking motivation. Many of the things you can practice on a daily basis include the way you think. Positive thinking is one of the biggest things you need to practice. Every time you feel negative about something, you need to pinch yourself and remember you are working on motivation. Positive thinking at all times will help you. See the good in everything.

The people you spend time together with have a big impact on you even if you do not think they do. When you surround yourself with positive and motivated people, you will feel the same way every day. The best thing you can do for you is hang around people who are supportive and believe in your goals. People who boost your spirit and your attitude are the best people you can have in your life. They will help create the motivation you need to meet goals and reach higher goals every day.

Daily motivational techniques need to be performed in order to feel great about achieving goals. As you begin working toward motivating yourself, you might find some of these methods difficult to perform. You might need to create a list of the things you need to do. These things may not come easily to you, and you will have to work hard toward all of these goals. Do not worry. After time you will find that your motivational techniques will come naturally to you, and you will no longer have to even try. You will be a motivated and positive person that most people love to be around too.

In conclusion, motivation is a journey that requires consistent effort and a positive mindset. By practicing positive thinking, surrounding yourself with supportive people, and implementing daily motivational techniques, you can cultivate the drive and enthusiasm needed to achieve your goals. Remember that motivation is not a static state but a dynamic process that evolves over time. Embrace the challenges and celebrate the victories along the way. With determination and a positive attitude, you can unlock your full potential and lead a fulfilling and motivated life.

~~~~~~~~~~~~~~~~~~~~~~~~~~~

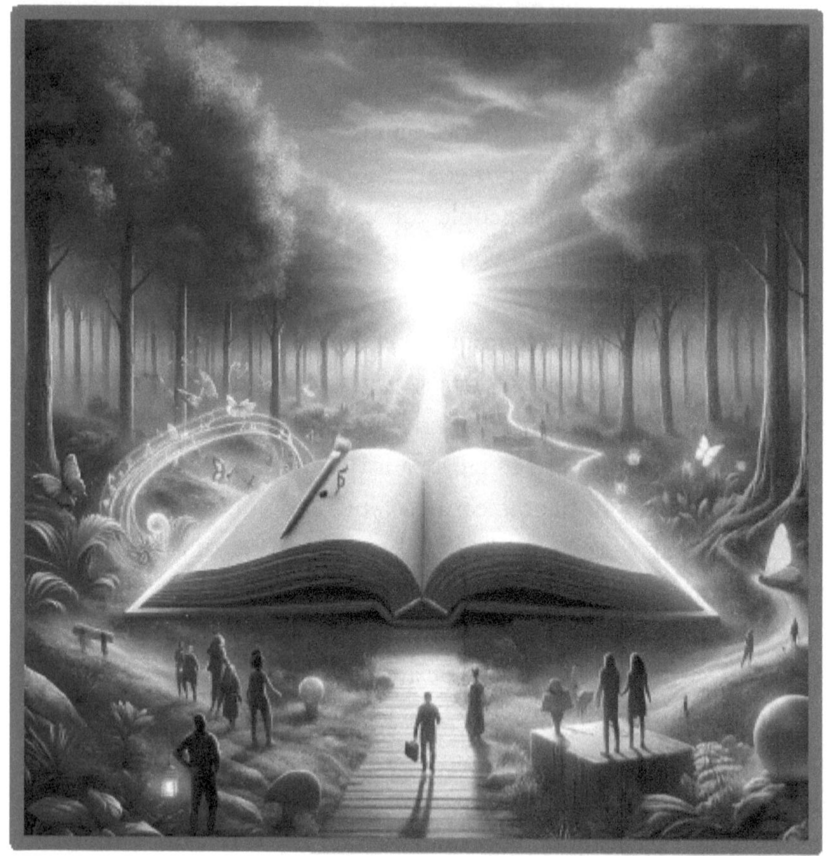

Epilogue:

As we reach the end of this journey on motivation, it is important to reflect on the lessons learned and the progress made. Motivation is not just a fleeting feeling but a driving force that propels us towards our goals and aspirations. It is the spark that ignites our passion and the fuel that keeps our engines running even when the road gets tough.

Throughout this book, we have explored various techniques and strategies to cultivate and maintain motivation. From setting clear goals
~~~~~~~~~~~~~~~~~~~~~~~~~~~

to surrounding ourselves with positive influences, each chapter has provided valuable insights into the art of staying motivated. But the journey does not end here. Motivation is a lifelong pursuit, and there will always be new challenges to face and new heights to reach.

As you move forward, remember that motivation is deeply personal. What works for one person may not work for another, so it is essential to find what resonates with you. Be open to experimenting with different approaches and be patient with yourself as you discover what truly motivates you.

One of the key takeaways from this book is the importance of self-awareness. Understanding your values, passions, and what drives you is crucial to maintaining motivation. Take the time to reflect on your experiences and learn from both your successes and failures. Every step, whether forward or backward, is a valuable lesson that contributes to your growth.

Another important lesson is the power of resilience. Motivation is not about avoiding obstacles but about having the courage and determination to overcome them. Embrace challenges as opportunities for growth and stay committed to your goals, even when the going gets tough.

As you continue on your motivational journey, remember to celebrate your achievements, no matter how small. Acknowledging your progress is a powerful motivator in itself and will inspire you to keep pushing forward.

Do not forget the significance of giving back and sharing your motivation with others. Helping others find their motivation can be incredibly rewarding and can further strengthen your own. Be a source of encouragement and inspiration to those around you, and you will find that your motivation will reach new heights.

In conclusion, the journey of motivation is ongoing and ever-evolving. It is a journey of self-discovery, resilience, and growth. As you close this book, take with you the lessons learned and the strategies that have resonated with you. Remember that motivation is within your reach, and with persistence and a positive attitude, you can achieve anything you set your mind to. Keep pushing forward, stay motivated, and embrace the endless possibilities that lie ahead.

~~~~~~~~~~~~~~~~~~~~~~~~~~
~~~~~~~~~~~~~~~~~~~~~~~~~~

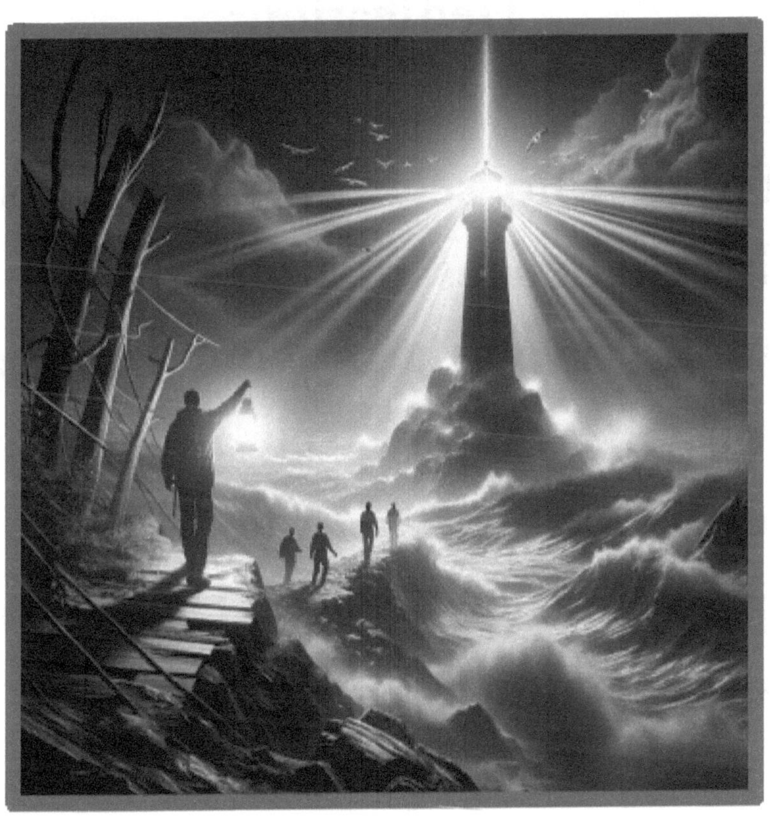

Dedication

To all who seek growth amidst the challenges of life—may this book serve as a beacon, guiding you towards self-awareness, resilience, and the joy of spreading positivity. Dedicated to the enduring spirit of every reader on their journey to becoming their best selves.

Always grateful,

Kevin James Joseph McNamara

~ ~ ~

#KevinJamesJoesphMcNamara
#KevinJJosephMcNamara
#KevinJJMcNamara

Staying Motivated
Daily Rituals to Stay Motivated!